LIVING IN THE LIGHT

LIVING IN THE LIGHT

Yoga for Self-Realization

DEEPAK CHOPRA, MD,
AND SARAH PLATT-FINGER

HARMONY
BOOKS · NEW YORK

Copyright © 2023 by Deepak Chopra

All rights reserved.
Published in the United States by Harmony Books,
an imprint of Random House, a division of
Penguin Random House LLC, New York.
HarmonyBooks.com
RandomHouseBooks.com

Harmony Books is a registered trademark, and the
Circle colophon is a trademark of Penguin Random House LLC.

Library of Congress Cataloging-in-Publication Data
is available upon request.

ISBN 978-0-593-23542-3
eBook ISBN 978-0-593-23543-0

Printed in the United States of America

Book design: Andrea Lau
Illustrations: Stephanie Singleton
Page 2 photograph: Makenna Colón
Cover design: Kathleen Lynch/Black Kat Design
Cover art: Benjavisa/iStock/Getty Images

10 9 8 7 6 5 4 3 2 1

First Edition

To everyone who aspires to live in the light

CONTENTS

PART I

By Deepak Chopra, MD

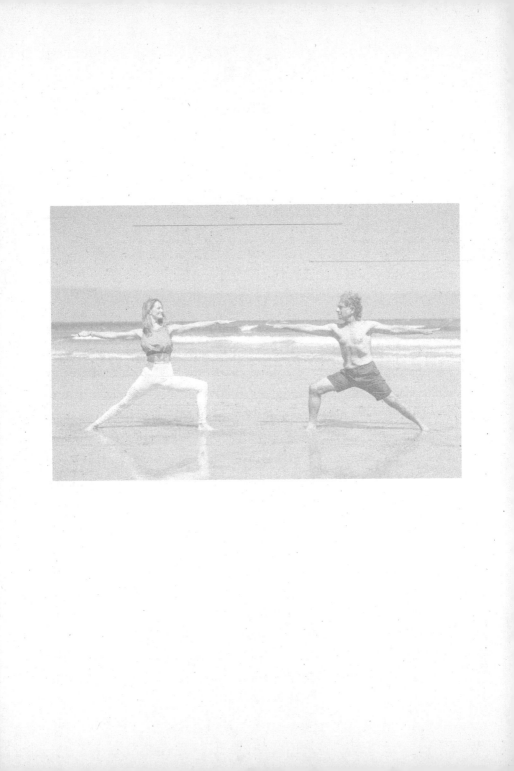

ROYAL YOGA AND THE LIGHT OF LIFE

Whatever you are doing to make your life better, Royal Yoga can bring you more of everything you want.

In that opening sentence lies the essence of this book, an immense promise that isn't just a matter of belief. For centuries in India, a path to fulfillment has been proven to work. In Sanskrit it is called Raja Yoga, *Raja* meaning "kingly," "royal," or simply "the highest." *Royal Yoga* is a splendid way to put it. My aim is to show you why and how the path of Royal Yoga is the highest and most important of all Yoga traditions, explaining everything in terms that apply to modern people and everyday life. As far as I know, this goal is unique; I've never found another book that accomplished it.

We are talking about personal transformation that reaches beyond any lifestyle you might choose to follow, beyond any approach to wellness and healing, beyond any faith or religion. Royal Yoga is universal and all-embracing.

The *Yoga* part of *Royal Yoga* needs a little clarification at the outset. The basic Sanskrit word *Yoga* simply means to yoke, join, or unite (the English word *yoke* can be directly traced back to its ancient roots). In my part of the book (Part I), when I talk about *Yoga*, I mean the *complete system* of Yoga, namely, the union of all aspects of life—physical, emotional, and spiritual. Only one part of the whole Yoga system contains the exercises that people learn in yoga class (I will put the exercise part in lowercase and refer to the system of Yoga with a capital Y). The system is often called "Yoga philosophy," but that phrase sells the whole vision short. In Royal Yoga, no aspect of existence is left out. Everyone is used to dividing life into distinct parts: mind, body, emotions, work, family, relationships, and so on. Those are handy divisions, of course. The experience of going to the doctor, the gym, or yoga class can all be put in the compartment labeled "body." Raising a child, going on a family vacation, and planning for retirement can all be placed in the compartment labeled "family." As natural as it feels to divide life in this way, this kind of compartmentalization creates a problem that cuts to the very heart of existence.

Royal Yoga holds that these compartments are false to the wholeness of life. There are hidden possibilities that you will never reach, an intensity of fulfillment you will never experience, when your life is chopped into separate pieces like a loaf of bread cut into neat slices. Imagine yourself going through certain rituals and habits of your day—you get up, eat breakfast, go to work, call friends, do things with your family, and so on. Take a moment to visualize some specific ways that might make your day more satisfying. Perhaps a friend tells you a piece of good news, you complete a project at work, or you watch your child or spouse smile at you and you feel a rush of love.

If you rewind these experiences and evaluate them through the prism of Yoga, each event might look the same on the surface. But if you practice Royal Yoga, what happens inside is transformed: You find that you are living in the light. The effect is all-embracing, because if there is life, there should be light.

What is the light? For some this is a vague spiritual term that connotes religion. A Christian might think of the phrase, "Don't hide your light under a bushel basket" or Jesus's declaration to his disciples, "You are the light of the world." In the rabbinical tradition of Judaism, the divine presence is Shechinah, which brings the light of God into the world when it permeates a devout or holy person. In many traditions, angelic beings are creatures of light, and saintly people emanate (physically or symbolically) a pure white light.

Royal Yoga transcends these religious connotations while embracing their deeper meaning. "Light" is pure awareness; it is the cosmic consciousness that creates and maintains the universe and everything in it. In practical terms, living in the light is about living consciously, and the ultimate goal in life is to live *only* in the light, having cast off every form of ignorance, pain, and suffering.

WHERE IS YOUR LIGHT?

Having read this far, you might be either skeptical or inspired. Something as all-embracing as Royal Yoga feels strange, at the very least. I'm not offering these concepts from the viewpoint of a true believer, because the vision of the Yoga tradition isn't a set of beliefs. It is based on experiences that everyone is already having. You already live in the light; you just don't live there all the time. Many people have experienced happiness, joy, and sometimes even pure bliss. But, on the flip side, there are dark experiences that bring confusion, pain, and suffering. Nonetheless, the light of life is always with you because light is your very nature, your true self.

Royal Yoga is unique because it seeks to make everyday life ideal. There is infinite bliss as the starting point, located in your true self. Whenever you experience less bliss, no bliss, or actual pain and suffering, only one thing changes: how close you are to the light. This concept defines the entire Yoga system, no matter how complex its traditions are in India. There are literally thousands of Yoga commentaries, and their intricacy can be mind-bending. But we can cut through the complexity by focusing on just one thing: living in the light.

It is vital to understand what the ideal life is, according to Royal Yoga. What makes its approach so natural is that nothing achieved through Royal Yoga is mystical or otherworldly. The self you experience today owes its most valued experiences to your true self, which is already whole and perfect.

The Ideal Life: The Gifts of Royal Yoga

1. Existence becomes blissful. You experience a joyful, energetic body; a loving, compassionate heart; an alert, vibrant mind; and lightness of being.
2. You control your mental activity. You can generate thoughts, feelings, and impulses that are evolutionary. You are the one who gives them meaning, and therefore the whole world as you perceive it has meaning.
3. You see everyday life as a lucid dream, incredibly vivid but an illusion. You can improve the dream without getting trapped in it.
4. Joy becomes the only measure of success because your essential nature is joy. It is the beginning and endpoint of every journey.
5. You understand what it means to thrive. You savor the diversity of life, which brings richness to your unfolding story.

6. You recognize that the point of arrival is always now. You can't move to where you are already standing—this is the experience of timelessness.

7. You recognize that you have no fixed identity. Your identity is unique but always evolving. It is your karmic story, but you don't need to be bound by it.

8. You recognize gratitude as the sanest response to existence. It is insanity to believe that existence is a problem.

9. You recognize that existence is lavish and abundant.

10. Grace becomes an everyday experience. It reveals itself by the perfect way that every experience fits together. Instead of brief glimpses of synchronicity, you live in total synchronicity.

Before we go any further, I'd like you to assess your experiences of the light. Nothing is more important than knowing how much the light has affected your life. Take the following self-assessment, and you will begin to know yourself much better than most people do.

Ten Ways to Be in the Light

Yoga asks you to identify entirely with the light, which doesn't happen all at once. The light is glimpsed, to begin with, in memorable experiences. Everyone has had them at one time or another. The list on the following pages includes the most important kinds of experiences.

To assess where you are right now, look at each statement and circle the response that applies to you. The time frame isn't critical—some experiences might be very recent; others very far back. The point is to recognize moments of heightened experience. There are no right or wrong responses. Just assess your experience as objectively as you can. When in doubt, choose the answer that first comes to mind.

1. **I have experienced bliss. (Examples: a peak experience of a joyful, energetic body; a loving, compassionate heart; an alert, vibrant mind; lightness of being.)**
    • Never
    • Rarely
    • Sometimes
    • Frequently
    • Don't know

2. **I feel in control of my mental experience—I can have positive, creative thoughts whenever I want.**
    • Never
    • Rarely
    • Sometimes
    • Frequently
    • Don't know

3. Life can feel like a dream, with something hidden from sight that is very real and yet mysterious.
    - Never
    - Rarely
    - Sometimes
    - Frequently
    - Don't know

4. Much more than material success, I measure my life by my level of happiness and joy.
    - Never
    - Rarely
    - Sometimes
    - Frequently
    - Don't know

5. I welcome a wide diversity of experiences—they give my life real richness.
    - Never
    - Rarely
    - Sometimes
    - Frequently
    - Don't know

6. **I live in the present moment, without reliving the past or anticipating the future.**
   - Never
   - Rarely
   - Sometimes
   - Frequently
   - Don't know

7. **I experience myself in the flow, adapting easily to new situations.**
   - Never
   - Rarely
   - Sometimes
   - Frequently
   - Don't know

8. **I experience gratitude.**
   - Never
   - Rarely
   - Sometimes
   - Frequently
   - Don't know

9. **I look upon life as abundant, offering untold possibilities for fulfillment.**
   • Never
   • Rarely
   • Sometimes
   • Frequently
   • Don't know

10. **I experience meaningful coincidences—they tell me that everything happens for a reason.**
   • Never
   • Rarely
   • Sometimes
   • Frequently
   • Don't know

ASSESSING YOUR ANSWERS

This questionnaire is about seeing yourself according to the quality of your inner life. Being in the light is what ties together these ten experiences. If you have a rich inner life, you will likely mark "Frequently" more than half the time. On the other hand, if you often answered "Never" or "Rarely," your inner life isn't fulfilling. The light has become blocked or obscured. Most people will fall somewhere in between the light and the dark. They are aware of their inner life, but don't turn to it as a great source of fulfillment.

For most of us, positive experiences come and go at will; we have little control over them. Fears, regrets, and painful memories seem to have a life of their own. Yoga teaches us to change the situation through the following steps, which will become second nature as the book unfolds:

You pay more attention to what is going on inside you.
You notice any experience of being in the light.
You value that experience.
You begin to focus more and more on the light, increasing
    it in your life.

Living in the light is the most natural way to live. It is easier to live more consciously than to continue experiencing things unconsciously, driven by habit, routine, old conditioning, and denial. The habit of being more conscious will emerge effortlessly and without pain and discomfort if you keep in mind that the best experiences in your life indicate that you have been living in the light all along, while struggling to get there.

THIRTY DAYS OF ROYAL YOGA

Living in the light can begin anytime you choose. The principles taught in Royal Yoga are not difficult to learn, and over the next thirty days we can cover all the major areas you need to understand. Traditionally, these areas are called the eight limbs, or *ashtangas*, of Yoga. We are going to treat them as eight stages of transformation.

Here is how a map of the journey looks. Our thirty-day journey is divided into six weeks, and each week gives you five days of participation—the weekend is your time off, to reflect upon and absorb everything you have learned.

I give the traditional Sanskrit names for the eight limbs, but you don't need to memorize them. What is important is the theme for each week, beginning with Social Intelligence in Week 1, Emotional Intelligence in Week 2, and so on. Living in the light involves awakening awareness, layer by layer, until you reach your source, the true self, which is the light of pure awareness.

Here's the whole program at a glance.

Week 1: Social Intelligence

(Stage of Transformation—Yama)

In the first week, you learn to find the light in your social world of family, work, and relationships. Royal Yoga considers this the outer shell of existence. You move through it with your own habits, rituals, likes, and dislikes. Your personality is your identity, which has been adapted from input and pressure from society. By bringing light and lightness to your social self, you prepare the way for the later stages of the journey.

Week 2: Emotional Intelligence

(Stage of Transformation—Niyama)

In the second week, you learn to bring light and lightness to your emotional life. Royal Yoga considers this stage to be more personal than the outer or social sphere, yet you are still involved with other people and your feelings toward them. When these feelings are purified, or brought into the light, you are not dependent on other people to trigger negative emotions in you. Victimhood and codependency are no longer the pitfalls they once were.

Week 3: Bringing the Light to Your Body

(Stage of Transformation—Asana)

In the third week, you learn to apply awareness to your body, bringing light and lightness to how you sense your body. Yoga considers the body to be a vehicle for consciousness. Just as a boat carries you across the ocean, your body carries you across the ocean of experience. Everyone is already on that journey. But, at a subtler level, your body is carrying you to wholeness and your true self. Royal Yoga teaches you to appreciate this aspect, which unites body and mind in a mutual relationship, the bodymind.

Week 4: Vital Energy

(Stage of Transformation—Pranayama)

In the fourth week, you learn to connect your breath with every state of the bodymind. Royal Yoga considers the breath to be the carrier of life energy. This energy animates your cells and organs, and brings vitality to your thoughts and moods. At a subtle level, breathing in and out is the bridge between all of creation "out there" and every experience "in here."

Week 5: Staying in the Light

(Stage of Transformation—Pratyahara)

In the fifth week, you learn to make the light your home base, no longer moving in and out of the light but always staying with it. Royal Yoga considers this the most significant transformation; it is like a second birth. A new existence opens. Realizing that you belong in the light, you now accept without a doubt that being completely whole and healed is your birthright.

Week 6: The Power of Attention

(Stages of Transformation—Dharana, Dhyana, Samadhi)

In the sixth week, the final three limbs are combined because they serve a single theme: the power of attention. Simply by paying attention to any thought, impulse, desire, or goal, you cause it to be fulfilled. Royal Yoga considers that knowledge is power, and the deeper your knowledge of consciousness and how it operates, the more power you possess. But this isn't knowledge in the sense of information or education. It is inner knowing that depends upon nothing but living in the light. The creative power of consciousness is revealed.

If you want to, you can jump directly to Week 1 of the journey, whose theme is Social Intelligence. But I'd like to expand a little more on why Yoga is distinct as a unique method of self-transformation.

"CHANGE YOURSELF, CHANGE THE WORLD"

Royal Yoga works—this has been proven over the centuries—and the reason it works is radical. In fact, the basic principle of the whole Yoga system is so revolutionary, it seems highly improbable that anyone would pursue it.

The principle is simply this: The world we think we live in is unreal. Like characters in a movie or a novel, we are living a fictional existence. Being unreal, this world we accept causes every kind of problem and suffering.

To return to your true self, you must understand how you got separated, or lost, in the first place. Yoga places the blame on *vrittis*, a Sanskrit word that literally means "whirlpools," but that Yoga uses to describe every form of mental disturbance. The most revered text in Yoga is Patanjali's *Yoga Sutras*, a text containing 195 aphorisms (sutras) outlining in authoritative fashion the entire scope of Yoga in theory and practice. No teaching is more important than the one concerning *vrittis*, which appears at the very outset of the book.

Here are the three opening sutras.

1. Now begins an exposition of Yoga.
2. Yoga is the cessation, or settling down, of the modifications of the mind (*vrittis*).
3. Then the knower is established in his own fundamental nature.

That's our entire journey in a nutshell. When the mind settles down into a quiet state, free from every kind of mental activity (*vritti*), the true self is revealed. This is straightforward as a path to the ideal life. The radical part, which is quite explosive, is packaged inside the word *vritti*, because, according to Yoga, every middle stage between you and your source is just a modification of the mind. The whole package of mind-made obstacles is known as *maya*, which is generally translated as "illusion," but includes distractions, deceptions, and mistaken thoughts and beliefs, all of which prevent us from experiencing the true self.

Is this a convincing way of looking at your life? It is undeniable that the mind creates suffering. The list of human troubles—war, crime, fear, depression, loneliness, suicide—is long and it belongs to no other living creature. It's the part about the world being unreal that stops everyone. "Walk in front of a bus," the skeptics scoff. "Then talk to me about how unreal everything is."

You might think there's no possible answer to that challenge. In fact, there is, and we'll come to it. Yoga isn't pointing to an illusion that will vanish in a puff of smoke. Buses, mountains, clouds, cities, and all other physical objects have their place, no matter what your worldview is. The unreality Yoga talks about runs deeper. It is a false foundation that undermines anything you try to build on it, like building a skyscraper on sand. No matter how beautiful, elaborate, and architecturally perfect the skyscraper is, resting it on a foundation of sand guarantees that it will topple.

We need Yoga if we want to put a secure foundation under our lives, because, if we don't, eventually we will pay a price in pain and suffering. If you want to base your life on reality instead of illusion, Yoga points to the bedrock of existence: consciousness. We do not actually live in the physical world, according to Yoga. We live in the world of experience, and every experience takes place in consciousness. Nothing is more basic.

The "real" reality is consciousness. That truth gives us a reliable starting point for being transformed. Next, we need the motivation to make us want to move forward. This is supplied by another radical idea: Change yourself, and you will change the world. You are the only agent of change that really counts. How do you create any change? By becoming more aware. The journey that takes us deeper into reality is worth taking, just because the more aware you are, the more things you can change—not just the world but your body, mind, emotions, beliefs, habits, indeed, anything you can think of.

Yoga is so radical, it overturns everything you and I have accepted since we were children. We've been chugging along year after year based on completely hollow beliefs and assumptions. Some beliefs matter more than others. These are known as "core beliefs," and when your core beliefs are wrong and misguided, trouble is always brewing—if not today, then in some worrisome future. To bring them closer to home, I'll list the core beliefs we all take personally.

FALSE CORE BELIEFS

I don't really matter. I am small, ordinary, and insignificant.

I deserve only so much love. At heart, I am probably unlovable.

Life hasn't been fair to me. That's because life is unfair.

If I don't look out for number one, no one else will.

There is much to fear in this world. Self-protection is very important.

If I show anyone that I am vulnerable, they will take advantage. I need to seem strong and independent.

The forces of Nature are all-powerful. I will be fortunate if some natural disaster doesn't befall me.

The universe is a vast, cold, empty void. The Earth and everyone on it are less than a speck of dust, a product of random events going back to the Big Bang.

These beliefs undermine everyone's life. They are ingrained in us early on, and they have sunk so deep into our sense of self that they hardly deserve a second glance.

If you accept the unreality that Yoga rejects, your core beliefs will seem completely logical. Look around you or listen to the twenty-four-hour news cycle. Isn't life unfair? Don't each of us deserve only a limited amount of love? Isn't the Earth a speck of dust floating in a cold, empty void?

As you'll see over the next thirty days, Royal Yoga holds out an ideal life based on a new set of core beliefs. These are literally the opposite of the false core beliefs we have all been mistakenly living by.

TRUE CORE BELIEFS

Your existence is based on an infinite field of consciousness. It is your source.

Your true self has access to infinite possibilities.

At your source, you are connected to infinite love and bliss.

Your true self is immune to fear, depression, aging, and death.

You are always completely safe. There is nothing to worry about.

You have no need to project an image of strength and independence.

You have no need to project any image at all.

The Earth and everything on it have a unique place in the tapestry of reality, woven by cosmic consciousness.

When people read these statements about an ideal life, they immediately assume they are merely someone else's beliefs, like the beliefs that underlie organized religion. Many would say that the entire issue of spirituality rests upon belief alone. It is impossible to accept Christianity unless you affirm the divinity of the resurrected Jesus, or so St. Paul declared in his letters to the early churches. It is impossible to accept Buddhism unless you affirm the Buddha's enlightenment and the existence of Nirvana. In the same way, to accept Yoga, you must affirm your own infinite standing in creation. From the perspective of everyday life, this seems like too much to swallow.

But nothing about the ideal life is a belief akin to religious beliefs. What's at stake is reality. Beliefs pertain to how you *feel* about reality. Yoga declares as a fact that every human being is embedded in a field of infinite potential. By squeezing our infinite potential down into small, manageable compartments, we are guilty only of being part of the mainstream of human beings. But Yoga doesn't care about the mainstream or about how you have lived in the past. In the worldview of Yoga, the infinite is always with us; in fact, it is our source. Nothing we do to squeeze our lives down to a manageable size has the slightest effect on reality, and the highest reality is what Royal Yoga is ultimately all about.

SOCIAL INTELLIGENCE

(Limb of Yoga: *Yamas*)

THIS PART OF THE JOURNEY

Royal Yoga begins by improving the social life you lead. Your interaction with other people reflects a lot about you. Inner forces are made visible, and it is these inner forces that dictate what happens to your social self, the self you show the world.

Very few people look at the reflections life gives them and see what they'd like to see. Even the people closest to us don't respond to us without adding their own slant—their own opinions, expectations, and beliefs—to what we say or do. We'll begin the journey of Royal Yoga by untangling the mixed reflections our social self is creating, because that's the only way to change how we relate to others and how they respond to us. We have a choice: Our social self can be radiant with light and lightness, or it can simply be an outer shell, created to serve our ego and burnish our self-image.

In short, Week 1 is about the story we are living and how to create a better story, one that reflects the levels of the self that are closer to our source.

MONDAY

Upgrading Your Story

Begin by silently repeating today's theme:

I create the peace that surrounds me.
I create the peace that surrounds me.

If your life story has been perfect up to now, there is no need to turn to Yoga to improve upon perfection. Everyone's personal story is created out of light and shadow. We defend ourselves against pain, which makes us fearful of the future, and against the past, which brings back painful moments. These self-imposed restraints are the focus of the first limb of Yoga, which Patanjali calls *yamas*, often translated to mean "guidelines" or "rules of conduct."

Note: I will make passing reference to Patanjali and his definitive work, the *Yoga Sutras*, but keep in mind that the traditional terminology isn't critical—only results are critical.

When you are aware of the self-imposed constraints you have placed on yourself, you can upgrade your story. As you progress limb to limb in Royal Yoga, the time will come when all stories you have bought into will melt away. But it is also true that you can't find the light when you are the one blocking it, and that's what unhappy stories do.

An upgraded story is easier to enjoy and therefore easier to escape from when the time comes. That's not a mystical statement. If you have a happy childhood, it is much easier to leave it behind than an unhappy childhood, which keeps returning to block future happiness.

Every spiritual tradition describes "right living" as an important goal, and Yoga agrees. The *yamas*, however, are not a series of ethical teachings. *Right living* in Yoga means "bringing in the light of awareness to decrease the things that block fulfillment." The five *yamas*, as interpreted for modern life, are the major keys to right living:

1. Treating everyone with peace and nonviolence.
2. Acting and speaking your own truth.
3. Acting unselfishly, without envy, greed, or covetousness.
4. Radiating a presence of purity and innocence.
5. Acting with self-reliance, neither clinging nor creating dependence in others.

Today is about the first *yama*, which asks you to live in peace with others. The goal is to relate peacefully with everyone. That is the first and most basic upgrade to your story.

Yoga's call for nonviolence is frequently misunderstood because people think they aren't spiritual unless they experience serenity and the peace that surpasses understanding. With that expectation in mind, they wind up patiently holding back their anger, even when it is justified, pretending to be more at peace than they really are, and feeling guilty about getting into arguments and engaging in conflict.

Inner peace is a wonderful state, but let's be clear: Our journey hasn't gotten there yet. The first limb of Yoga is about social tactics—using your intelligence to bring more light and lightness into the story you are now living.

The tactics for creating a peaceful life are available to everyone, as follows:

THE PRACTICES OF PEACE

Don't create stress for yourself and others.

Look for areas of agreement instead of areas of discord.

Take responsibility for your own anger and resentment. Don't unleash them on other people.

Get out of the habit of blaming others.

Be aware of your impulse to judge, criticize, and get offended. Don't indulge in the impulse whenever possible.

Distance yourself from hostile people and hostile situations.

If you adopt these practices, you won't be leading a saintly life. You will have succeeded in right living, however, which, at this stage is a huge step in your evolution.

Exercise

Take time to look over the practices of peace listed above, and honestly ask yourself how well you are practicing them. Social intelligence is a skill, and, like all skills, it can be learned. Learning doesn't come all at once but in pieces, so take a single strategy from the list, and set your own learning curve. Anger is a good one to begin with, because, along with fear, it is one of the two basic negative emotions.

Yama asks you to be responsible for your anger, not to pass it along, unleash it on the unwary, or channel it as blame toward another. To make practical use of this *yama*, start following right tactics.

When you feel yourself getting angry, pause and stop at the first sign that you are losing your temper.

Be with the impulse.

Sit in your awareness for just a moment.

Pausing to be aware is a powerful way to defuse any self-defeating be-havior. If after pausing your anger comes out anyway, you have still made a start. When you are calmer, ask if your outburst made the situation better. If you can see clearly that it didn't—it probably made the situation worse—you have taken another step toward inner awareness.

Yoga teaches that all your behaviors are subject to your control. If you want the practices of peace to bring peace under your control, follow the two steps I mentioned for anger. Namely, pause when you find yourself not acting peacefully. Then, if you did not manage to control that behavior, pause and ask yourself if you improved the situation or made it worse.

Even though I will be unfolding Yoga one week at a time, its teachings are meant for a lifetime. The practices of peace work. They will definitely upgrade your story. Don't pressure yourself to adopt them. Just make them part of your awareness as you grow in social intelligence.

TUESDAY

Living Your Truth

Begin by silently repeating today's theme:

I trust the truth to show me the way.
I trust the truth to show me the way.

The second *yama* is about speaking and acting from our own truth. The social self is very good at bending the truth. Many of us have practiced "go along to get along," which taught us not to say what's on our minds. We fear retaliation if we tell certain people the painful truth about their short-comings. We cringe at the notion that someone else will embarrass or humiliate us by exposing our own faults. The second *yama* addresses the messy relationship all of us have with the truth.

The problem begins with the difference between two kinds of truth—relative truth and absolute truth. When you live in the light, absolute truth upholds you. For example, it is an absolute truth that love is eternal, that life is infinitely abundant, and that life is meant to be lived without struggle. When you are merged with your true self, absolute truth is who you are.

But your social self deals in relative truths. Relative truth causes more trouble than it resolves; therefore, you need to use the right tactics that apply to this part of your story. Relative truth is defined by the situation you find yourself in. A parent scolding a child for misbehaving isn't in the same situation as an adult scolding another adult. In the first case, parental guidance truthfully teaches right from wrong. In the second case, the scolding is an affront, because one adult doesn't have the right to impose his moral values on another adult.

Relative truth isn't stable or reliable. It is constantly open to disagreement. Being certain that you are right and someone else is wrong creates endless hostility in traffic jams, religion, politics, and family life. Yet each person justifies their participation in the hostilities by feeling that they have truth on their side. To upgrade your story in this area, Royal Yoga provides essential tactics to increase social intelligence.

THE PRACTICES OF TRUTH

Abandon the certainty that you are always right.

Allow the possibility that everyone has their own truth.

Hold on to your truth in silence. Don't rush to broadcast it.

Don't make other people wrong.

Realize that your truth exists to bring light into your life and those around you.

Don't use "I'm only telling the truth" as a cover for blame, criticism, and discord.

When your truth is compatible with the light, it will create no problems for you. When your truth is a disguise for the desire to wound, criticize, and blame other people, you are not even practicing relative truth—you are lying to yourself instead.

Exercise

Glance over the list of practices for living your truth. Take an honest look at how well you are following these practices. The first step, as noted earlier, is to pause and stop yourself from following an impulse that would make the situation worse. The second step is to reflect afterward if your response helped the situation.

For example, imagine that you are talking to a friend or family member whose beliefs you strongly disagree with. The most sensitive topics tend to be the familiar ones: religion, politics, and money. You feel an impulse to set this person straight, acting out of the certainty that you know the truth. This certainty is a sure sign that you are using relative truth for the wrong ends. There is no possibility that you will set the other person straight. You will be creating resistance and hostility instead. The stress level for both of you will rise.

How do you know that those negative reactions will be the outcome? Social intelligence tells you so. Bashing someone over the head with your truth is a perfect example of doing more of what never worked in the first place. By holding back, you are choosing a higher truth, and the higher truth is that bringing light to any situation begins by not increasing the darkness.

WEDNESDAY

Being Yourself

Begin by silently repeating today's theme:

I embrace the wholeness of myself.
I embrace the wholeness of myself.

The third *yama* is about acting unselfishly, without envy, jealousy, greed, or covetousness. What makes this guidance hard to follow is that we are constantly comparing our stories to someone else's. The rich, powerful, and gifted seem to exist to fuel envy, and when we are driven by social climbing and ambition, these motivations typically come from a desire not to be seen as inferior or to be left behind. As a result, "I want your story instead of mine" is easier to indulge than upgrading your own story.

Royal Yoga teaches that stories are just temporary phases. The things you envy and covet are not the values of the true self. You can choose to envy the rich and famous, and this might provide you with motivation to claw and compete for your chance at the golden ring. But in your fierce focus and determination, you will lose sight of the wholeness of life.

While we use the word *wholeness* to refer to everything from whole foods to holistic medicine, Yoga has a unique view of it. The Yogic view is that you are already whole but don't realize it. Instead of striving to overcome your inner struggle, along with the beliefs and conditioning of a lifetime, Royal Yoga advises only one thing, and that thing is to be yourself, because no other behavior will open the way to realizing your true self.

The practices of the *yamas* are like a testing ground to determine if Yoga's view of wholeness literally works. By practicing the third *yama*, you do away with envy, greed, and covetousness simply by being yourself, moving away from the habits that keep you from knowing who you really are.

THE PRACTICES OF BEING YOURSELF
Stop comparing yourself to others.
Don't depend on other people to validate you.
Set aside the criticism and judgments of others.
Get beyond self-judgment.
Accept who you are and appreciate what you have to offer.
Give everyone the space to be themselves.
Assume that all people, in their essence, are whole.

The key to these practices is to live without comparing yourself to anyone else. In classic Yoga this *yama* is specifically about not being envious and covetous. I've expanded the theme for modern life, in which mass media floods us with reasons to feel inadequate because we aren't as rich, beautiful, smart, or talented as someone else; therefore, we feel the need to acquire more and more of the things we lack. Endless consumerism offers substitutes for embracing who we are. Craving the next iPhone, a bigger SUV, more premium channels on your smart TV, and all the rest of the flashy material things around us is a hollow surrogate for the true self.

Royal Yoga isn't telling you to look at your present life and call it perfect—the *yamas* are all about upgrading your story. Approach your life with an attitude of "I am enough in myself," instead of an attitude of insecurity and lack. Social intelligence tells us that such a negative starting point won't bring a better life; it only makes your present life less rewarding.

Exercise

You cannot be yourself if you are constantly distracted. Today's exercise is about becoming more aware of those times when you are stressed, worried, overwhelmed, confused, or distracted in any way. The moment you notice that you are feeling any of these things, find a moment to be alone in a quiet place.

Take a few deep breaths, close your eyes, and center your attention in the region of your heart. Easily follow your breathing as you breathe in and out. Don't try to control or suppress any thoughts that arise. Don't try to change anything. Just be easy with the moment as it presents itself because that's the basis for a life in wholeness.

This simple practice of centering yourself will reappear over and over again on our journey. No matter which limb of Yoga you are focused on, it is crucial for the experience to be natural and easy. Nothing is more natural or easier than being yourself. Your sense of self is your lifelong companion, and it will bring immense rewards as you begin to realize that the self you sense is the true self.

THURSDAY

The Value of Innocence

Begin by silently repeating today's theme:

I treat every day like a new world.
I treat every day like a new world.

The fourth *yama* is about radiating a presence of purity and innocence. The contrast with modern life could hardly be more glaring. As time moves inexorably forward from the moment we are born, innocence is left behind. Our experiences teach us about the risks and obstacles in life, we stop trusting automatically and begin to distrust just as automatically. Most people would agree with this thumbnail sketch, but Royal Yoga pushes back. Reality is timeless, and the things we lose, such as innocence and trust, shouldn't be lost. They fade from our lives because we buy into a scheme that everyone agrees on, the scheme that idealizes youth and dreads the ravages of time.

Right now, you can stop buying into the illusion that your life is ruled by the clock and the calendar. The light is always present; every day is a new beginning; and innocence can always be reborn. Adopt those principles, and your behavior will follow suit.

As applied to your social self, innocence involves a set of practices, just as all the *yamas* do.

THE PRACTICES OF INNOCENCE

Don't bring old expectations to new situations.
Don't fear the present because of bad experiences in your past.
Practice trust, including the ability to trust yourself.

Be open to other people as your default, rather than being defensive or suspicious of them.

Be attuned to the mood of people around you. Don't impose your own mood on them.

In place of trying to control other people and the events of the day, give them space to unfold the way they want to.

As with the other *yamas*, these principles are based on social intelligence. You are not aiming to change your inner beliefs and habits. That's why the word *tactics* applies. Yet there are deeper levels to the *yamas*, and one level is about the proper use of energy. The connection with innocence isn't obvious, so let me explain.

Royal Yoga teaches that energy you expend during the day is yours to control and, as you become better at controlling it, more energy is provided. This applies to every kind of energy—physical, mental, and emotional. A good example is the energy of love. Falling in love is a disorganized state, known as "infatuation." When you are infatuated, nothing matters but the beloved, and all your energies are directed at your beloved, including sexual energy. When you are caught up in infatuation, the other aspects of daily life get neglected. At the opposite end of the spectrum is a loveless existence. None of the joy and vibrancy of love is present; the other aspects of life get all your attention.

Yet there is a stage of mature love in which a steady flow of both loving and sexual energy is present. Two people share in the contentment and trust that mature love brings, and their love evolves into deeper levels of caring and appreciation. The connection to innocence happens because both people are open to the other, not building up old resentments, hurts, disagreements, and a feeling of "same old, same old."

Innocence is the same as having no agenda. Without falling in love, you can treat everyone in your life with openness and appreciation. That's a mark of social intelligence, because you are using your physical, mental, and emotional energy without exhausting yourself on the one hand or being ruled by inertia on the other. In classic Yoga, the fourth *yama* is associated with sexual chastity, but for modern people, the real issue is not sexual innocence and purity but the right use of every kind of energy.

Exercise

Make a list of the people and situations where you are wasting your energy or using it ineffectually. The telltale signs are that your efforts are getting you nowhere; you feel exhausted; frustration is always present; and you keep trying too hard without results. Almost always there is also a buildup of low expectations and the memory of past failure and frustration.

Your list might include a family member who never does their chores, a child you constantly worry about, or a coworker who keeps demanding your time in trivial ways.

Now look at the person or situation from the viewpoint of your energy and how you expend it. Use the categories of physical, mental, and emotional energy. For instance, maybe a friend of yours is consistently late, and this inconsiderate behavior causes you a lot of irritation. Every time the behavior is repeated, that leaves you out of sorts, feeling drained and regretting setting up the get-together.

But it is important to realize that your energy is not being drained or exploited by someone else. It is being drained and exploited by you.

Your response has stopped being open, and you are pursuing, however silently, an agenda of being long-suffering that complements your friend's agenda of inconsideration. There is always a better way to deal with your own energy so that no agenda is involved. Look at the practices listed for the fourth *yama* and take the first step to applying at least one of them. Measure your success by how your own energy level improves—that's the goal of this *yama*.

FRIDAY

The Joy of Letting Go

Begin by silently repeating today's theme:

I feel no need to cling or grasp.
I feel no need to cling or grasp.

The fifth *yama* is about acting with self-reliance, neither clinging nor creating dependence in others. Not clinging is synonymous with letting go. Everyone has experienced finally letting go after the struggle of holding on has exhausted itself. The moment of letting go brings a sigh of relief. A burden has been lifted, and you are free to move on. The experience of letting go is so gratifying, you wonder why people do the opposite, holding on to grudges, resentments, bad relationships, self-defeating habits, and so on. Royal Yoga devotes the last *yama* to non-clinging because the inability to let go is age-old and has many tentacles.

Your social self has been trained to adopt the ego's agenda, which can be simply stated as "more for me." We grasp, cling, and hold on as a reflex, our default for getting more money, more love, more pleasurable experiences to ward off the threat of loss. In psychological terms, the result of clinging, when it happens in a relationship, is codependency. Two people cling to each other, even though what the ego wants—love, sexual gratification, security, and respect—isn't being delivered anymore. The habit of clinging has taken over without anything positive to show for it. "But at least we stayed together" is the rationale behind codependent relationships.

Royal Yoga's aim is to break the habit of clinging, whether it is in the early or late stages. Social intelligence teaches that when you have your own space and you give space to others, everyone benefits. The practices of non-clinging spring from this realization.

THE PRACTICES OF NON-CLINGING

Ask for the space you need from other people. Give others the same space before they have to ask.

Don't encourage someone to cling to you out of pity or superiority.

Practice self-reliance and independence.

Take responsibility for your life, finding solutions on your own.

Avoid relationships where one person dominates the other.

Drop the need to control.

Don't be grasping about money and possessions. Choose generosity whenever you can.

If you apply these practices in daily life, a change starts to occur. You catch yourself clinging in ways that are not productive and most of the time are self-defeating. It is nearly impossible to follow the ego's agenda of "more for me" without at the same time clinging to what you acquire, whether it is money and possessions or status and family.

Relationships form the acid test. Social intelligence is realistic. It recognizes that most people have a strong streak of dependency. They are more than willing to be led by a stronger, more dominant person. They feel too weak or insecure to practice self-reliance. In the face of this reality, many relationships are about finding the "missing piece." Two people find mutual support because they supply what the other person is lacking.

Missing-piece relationships are perhaps the most common, and they can bring a sense of security and belonging. The pitfall is the illusion of being whole. Two incomplete people do not make a whole, and wholeness is the goal of Yoga. Yet it is also possible that with loving support, two people can encourage each other to evolve and fulfill the wholeness that is found in the true self.

Exercise

The temptation to cling to someone else is strong when we feel incomplete in ourselves. Take a look at your spouse or partner (if you're single, choose your closest friend or family member) and list the ways in which you feel he or she is better than you. Is this person smarter, more creative, more popular, or a higher earner? Do they seem more self-confident than you or more successful at getting along with others?

Your list shows you where you have a missing piece, a hole in your self-esteem. Now think of ways to fill these holes yourself. Begin by not clinging to the other person. It is certainly good to admire your spouse or friend for their positive qualities. But you aren't a sponge that can soak those qualities up. Earning them for yourself is the only way.

What you are looking for in any relationship is mutual respect, first from your spouse or friend, but also from others, who might be tempted to think, "He's smart enough for both of us" or "She's got more than enough money for two." Inequality in money, job success, and social standing destabilizes a mutual relationship. Think about how you can find something valuable that you can contribute; it should be something that makes you feel more self-sufficient and worthy.

You don't have to even the balance by competing—this tactic rarely works. Let your partner or friend bask in the qualities that are special about them, while developing in yourself the qualities that make you special. The values that matter most are love, compassion, creativity, service, joy, intelligence, personal evolution, and self-awareness. All of them belong to your true self, and when you pursue these values as a social self, you begin to connect more closely to your true self, which is your source.

ADVANCED EXPLORATION

If you want to go more deeply into classic Yoga, there are many sources of information about the *yamas*, beginning with all the free information online. Look under the Sanskrit names for the *yamas*, which are given below with their traditional translations.

Ahimsa: Non-violence
Satya: Truthfulness
Asteya: Non-covetousness
Brahmacharya: Sexual restraint
Aparigraha: Non-grasping, non-clinging

EMOTIONAL INTELLIGENCE

(Limb of Yoga: *Niyamas*)

THIS PART OF THE JOURNEY

In Week 1 we dealt with your social self, which is how you present yourself to the world and other people. In Week 2 we move on to your emotional self, which relates to you personally and privately. Only you know how you feel and what makes you happy or unhappy. The journey of Royal Yoga is about moving ever closer to your true self. Every step of the way makes the light brighter and removes another layer of mental obstacles (*vrittis*) that block the light. These two steps never change.

The second limb of Yoga outlines the practices known as *niyamas*. They are complementary to *yamas*, since both involve "right living." But the five *niyamas* are subtler and more intimate. Everyone's emotions are a tangle of positive and negative feelings, which make them a perfect area for learning how to distinguish the light from the darkness. This happens when we develop our emotional intelligence. Everyone has emotional intelligence, but it's usually at a level not very far advanced from childhood. Our emotions come and go without any sort of conscious control.

Before you can control your emotions, you first need to understand what *control* means. It doesn't mean suppressing, pushing down, or denying those feelings you find undesirable and don't want to experience. Instead, emotional control, as Yoga sees it, means finding the core of bliss that is your true self and returning to it. The five *niyamas* give you the skills to accomplish this.

MONDAY

Purified Emotions

Begin by silently repeating today's theme:

I experience the light through my emotions.
I experience the light through my emotions.

In most people's lives, their emotions control them, rather than the other way around. The sharp rise in anxiety and depression over the past few decades provides stark evidence of this. It therefore sounds strange, even unbelievable, that Royal Yoga asks us to bring our emotions under control. Fear, worry, and anxiety should not be allowed to roam the mind at will. Grief and sadness should not overwhelm us to the point of paralysis and helplessness.

These conditions come about, according to Yoga, because of impressions made on the emotional self. Emotional wounds are just as real as physical ones, but the impressions Yoga describes, known as *samskaras*, are invisible, and quite often we have no memory of how or when they occurred.

Even without knowing where they came from, these holdovers from your past are the obstacles that block the light. In emotional terms, the light is experienced as bliss. When your emotional self is in direct contact with your true self, you will experience bliss as a normal state. The five *niyamas* give you the skills to make that connection. Each skill strengthens your emotional intelligence, as follows:

1. Observing mental hygiene, which purifies the emotions
2. Learning to be contented, self-accepting, and accepting of other people
3. Transforming old, outworn emotional habits
4. Clearly understanding that your true self is real, tangible, and powerful
5. Recognizing your higher reality and surrendering to it

Royal Yoga is based on the power of consciousness, which includes the power to heal the past. If your emotional life is spent entirely in the present, the past is automatically healed—you don't return there anymore. The trick isn't how to be in the present moment—you are there anytime you focus on whatever is before you, whether you're boiling an egg, bringing a child home from school, or meeting a deadline at work.

The trick is to remain in the present. The mind is thrown out of present-moment awareness by all kinds of distractions. The *niyamas* are concerned with emotional distractions. The worst of these are negative emotions that arise spontaneously, including fear, worry, shame, guilt, anger, and their nasty relations.

Therefore, the first *niyama* is about purifying your emotions to rid them of these toxic distractions. Until it is distorted by *vrittis*, awareness, by its very nature, is unblemished, or pure. How does this relate to emotions?

Your emotional self is where old wounds are stored as impressions. Whatever makes these impressions dark, such as humiliations, shame, and guilt from the past, are the impurities that need healing.

THE PRACTICES FOR EMOTIONAL HEALING

Favor your positive emotions.

Reject the memory of old hurts.

Face your feelings honestly without denying or repressing them.

Realize that the past is gone, except as an illusion of memory.

Pursue friendships that accentuate positive emotions.

Be easy with yourself, not putting pressure on yourself to change.

Look at your emotions with a measure of detachment. Don't overly indulge or exaggerate them.

Return to bliss as often as you can.

Untrain your old habitual emotional responses.

All these practices are based on bliss as a permanent reality and distorted awareness as temporary. What follows is that our negative emotions are learned responses. Somewhere in our past we started favoring, usually in small ways, being sad, helpless, worried, victimized, or depressed, just to name the most common emotional habits. These small beginnings began to cascade the more we relied on them. What started out as defensive and protective behavior reaches a tipping point. (Passivity, for example, is a psychological form of playing possum, defending yourself by not attracting attention.) After that, you have trained your emotional self to use this learned behavior all the time.

In that context, the purity called for in the first *niyama* is a clean slate, and the practices involved are reminders that you can clean the slate—

whatever is learned can be unlearned. The opposite of purity is toxicity, and the first *niyama* can be expressed as freeing yourself from toxicity.

THE PRACTICES FOR CLEARING TOXINS

Expose yourself to uplifting people and experiences.

Go out into Nature as much as possible.

Get 8 to 9 hours of steady good sleep every night.

Avoid physical toxins, such as alcohol, drugs, and tobacco.

Keep away from friends and family with persistent negative attitudes.

Work in a happy, positive environment.

Get enough physical activity every day to feel flexible and active.

Your body has natural mechanisms for detoxifying itself. This has long been recognized physically through the action of organs like the kidneys, which remove toxins from the blood. But there is a mental and psychological connection, too, because it was discovered that the brain uses sleep to clear away toxic debris from the previous day.

The first *niyama* goes a level deeper, to the spiritual state of purity, which is based on pure awareness. But *deeper* also means "expanded," because Yoga teaches that awareness is the ultimate healer, no matter at what level it occurs.

Exercise

With pen and paper in hand, go over the two lists of practices for emotional healing and clearing toxins. Rate yourself on how well you think you are doing in both areas. Take one of your strongest points and write down ways you can expand it. Having done that, write down your weakest point and write down how to improve it.

Perhaps your weakest point is that you let old memories of past hurts return too much. You can untrain yourself by adopting the habit of looking these memories in the eye and silently saying, "I don't need you anymore." You can sit and center yourself in a simple breathing meditation until the memory subsides. You can get up and take a few moments to stretch and move around, which is often quite effective in making negative thoughts dissipate naturally.

Your strongest points are likely to be much easier to address—simply do more of the things that inspire you and you will naturally bring out an experience of bliss. So why engage in this exercise? Writing down your strong points reminds you not to take them for granted and forget to reinforce them.

TUESDAY

Finding Self-Acceptance

Begin by silently repeating today's theme:

Being myself brings contentment.
Being myself brings contentment.

The second *niyama* is about learning to be contented, self-accepting, and accepting of other people. A basic teaching in Royal Yoga is that you cannot reach your true self without making peace with your other selves first. The easiest way to understand this is by looking at the opposite. If you are discontented with your emotional life, your discontent will nag at you about the same emotional issues over and over again. Like a magnet, your mind will be attracted back to your unresolved anger, resentment, envy, and fear. The impressions of the past (*samskaras*) exist to attract your attention, not to hurt you but to motivate you to seek change.

Discontent is not enough on its own to drive a person forward on the spiritual path. You cannot get beyond emotional pain by dwelling on it; that's a basic insight of emotional intelligence. The problem is that discontent only serves to fuel more discontent. There has to be the added element provided by the second *niyama*, which focuses on finding contentment and self-acceptance here and now.

THE PRACTICES FOR SELF-ACCEPTANCE

Remind yourself of your own goodness and worth. Reject any opinion
   to the contrary, either from yourself or from others.
Find something every day to be contented with.
Reinforce your happy experiences.
Don't dwell on your unhappy experiences.
Be around people who have high self-esteem.
Choose activities that make you feel good about yourself.
Be vigilant that you don't fall into false self-worth (the symptoms are
   vanity, egotism, pride, arrogance, and boasting).
Don't make other people feel small so that you can feel bigger.

The underlying teaching behind all these practices is that your emotional self exists to bring fulfillment. You aren't here to be important, successful, and respected while feeling miserable inside. You aren't here to pursue pleasure or to distract yourself from pain. Even though your emotional self isn't your true self, it should mirror your true self, which is silently sending you impulses of bliss and total self-acceptance.

The *niyamas* are also defined by what *you shouldn't do* if your aim is right living. Being aware of what not to do is just as productive as knowing the practices for self-acceptance. Emotional intelligence contains both. The opposite of self-acceptance is low self-esteem, so this is the area to focus on.

WAYS YOU LOWER YOUR SELF-ESTEEM

Comparing yourself unfavorably to other people.

Reminding yourself of your shortcomings.

Condemning all your mistakes, however trivial.

Setting up an ideal of perfection that you will never attain.

Being unreasonable in the demands you place on yourself.

Holding on to old experiences of guilt and shame.

Pretending to be better than you actually think you are.

Deprecating yourself in moments of false modesty.

I've offered many specifics in these two lists, yet emotional intelligence isn't difficult to come by, nor is self-acceptance. Just keep in mind that your emotional life isn't the be-all and end-all of existence. By their nature, emotions rise and fall. If you accept this basic fact—that your feelings are transient and can be mercurial, even on your best days—half the job of self-acceptance is done. You have achieved a measure of detachment, which allows you not to be so consumed by your feelings, especially the negative ones; they are events in your mental activity, not aspects of your essential true self.

You are never going to have a blissful emotional life by struggling with your emotions or trying to escape them, either. This is one area where allowing life to unfold naturally, without interference, is very effective.

Exercise

The single most important practice for contentment is not to resist the flow of life. In other words, take things as they come. The opposite of this is to offer resistance. Pause to reflect on the people you tend to resist in various ways. Often, they are the people who are closest to you, whether family members, colleagues, or even friends. Consider the kinds of resistance that are casually practiced. They include:

Bickering and arguments
Unresolved disagreements
Rejection
Ridicule
Resentment
Feeling either superior or inferior
Pushing people away
Expressing a lack of respect
Nagging
Indulging in petty criticisms

Emotional intelligence teaches that resisting others contributes to your own lack of contentment and self-acceptance. One way of increasing contentment in your life is to back down from unnecessary habitual resistance. Try using the principle of opposites. For instance, if you realize that you can be highly critical, begin practicing criticism's opposite: praise. Instead of pointing out someone's flaws or complaining, take a breath and offer a word of admiration or encouragement. Using this simple tactic becomes your way of contributing to the flow of life.

WEDNESDAY

The Fire of Transformation

Begin by silently repeating today's theme:

I allow the light to create transformation.
I allow the light to create transformation.

The third *niyama* is about transforming your old emotional habits. Habits block the light by forcing you to react automatically without consciously being in control. In classic Yoga, the lasting impressions that rob us of choice are like seeds that must be burned away. The burning is done by awareness itself, using the light's ability to purify the mind. It is also taught that the fire of transformation burns away ignorance. The point here is that the obstacles that keep us from living in the light are frozen bits of consciousness. Therefore, only consciousness can melt them away.

Old forms must be destroyed to make room for the new. This makes perfect sense emotionally. If you are consumed with resentment about a failed relationship, a bad boss, or an unfair monetary loss, you can't move on until the emotion you are stuck in is dissipated.

There is considerable misunderstanding about how the process works, however, and words like *fire*, *destroy*, and *burn* can mislead someone into thinking that some kind of violence is involved. In many religious traditions the ritual of mortifying the flesh had the intention of purifying the spirit, using the body's pain as the fire. Fortunately, such rituals are irrelevant to modern life. Simply by focusing your awareness, you can begin to burn away the *vrittis* that block your true self. It takes dedication to achieve transformation. Focus is a necessity.

We are all familiar with how focus works whenever we become absorbed in a game or hobby. Focusing for hours at a time without feeling any strain is entirely natural. Royal Yoga teaches that experiences like these are gateways to the true self. Becoming absorbed in the moment comes naturally, so the only change is that you focus inwardly. Then you can allow your awareness to do what it already wants to do, which is to find the light. The practices of the third *niyama* expand upon this basic insight.

THE PRACTICES OF SELF-TRANSFORMATION

Have an interest in finding your true self.

Enjoy going inside.

Value every experience of being in the light.

Don't look for fulfillment in the outside world.

Make conscious choices, instead of following unconscious habit and routine.

Welcome change, instead of resisting it.

See every experience as a mirror of yourself.

Regularly meditate.

Take the opportunity for "in time" and "down time" every day.

These are all gentle practices, but the profoundest transformation is gentle. Unlike our struggle to improve ourselves, the essence of transformation is to allow the light to do all the work. This is the law of least effort. What you are aiming for is a series of revelations, insights, and "Aha!" moments. They signal that change is at hand. Only the light can deliver these transformative experiences. Your ego and a burning desire to get rid of the things you dislike about yourself cannot do the job. You will be surprised at how steadily revelation comes once you get out of the way and allow the focus of awareness to develop of its own accord.

Exercise

The key to transformation is getting out of the way, which happens to be the opposite of what most people do when they desire change. They struggle, push themselves, and fight against frustration. (A good example of how futile those tactics are is revealed in the dismal fact that only 2 percent of dieters, in their struggle to lose weight, succeed in keeping off 5 pounds for two years.)

You can turn this pattern around in two ways. First, look honestly at an area of your life where you have struggled and resolve not to keep doing what never worked in the first place. Second, find enjoyable ways to meet yourself "in here." As alluded to earlier, seek some "in time" and "quiet time" every day. Stillness concentrates the light, while chaos scatters it. Become accustomed to the comfort of being in communion with yourself. Once this becomes your new habit, you are getting out of the way, setting the stage for the process of transformation as it is really designed to work.

THURSDAY

Tracking Your True Self

Begin by silently repeating today's theme:

I reflect on my true self to bring it closer.
I reflect on my true self to bring it closer.

The fourth *niyama* calls for clearly understanding that your true self is real, tangible, and powerful. The word *self* is one of the most important in Yoga, and most people will have no trouble seeing that they have a social self and an emotional self. Much more foreign is the notion that everyone has a true self, hidden like a jewel in the stormy activity of the mind.

Various interpretations speak of this *niyama* as self-reflection, but it matters deeply whether you are reflecting on a self you can trust and have faith in. Without a doubt, we don't fully trust our emotions. We feel them, sometimes strongly, but they are temporary, changeable, and fickle. It is baffling why this *niyama* would ask you to reflect upon the swirling whirl-pool of your emotions.

The key is that self-reflection enables you to stand aside and not become so involved in your emotions. Think about a moviegoer who sits entranced by an adventure film or a romantic comedy on the screen, and yet who doesn't know that he's watching a movie or, worse, that movies even exist.

We are all that moviegoer to some degree or other. Entranced by the movie we are living, we don't realize the illusory nature of what we are watching, and, worse still, we don't realize that everything we observe is the play of consciousness. Self-reflection clears up this confusion and therefore points us toward our true self.

THE PRACTICES OF SELF-REFLECTION

Keep in mind that you are here to evolve.

Don't get stuck in emotional habits.

Place a high value on experiences that reflect your true self (e.g., love, compassion, beauty, insight, creativity, and mental clarity).

Don't add to the drama around you.

Resist buying into other people's drama.

Avoid immersing yourself in news stories about catastrophes,
    disasters, and looming threats.
Realize that worry isn't productive.
Reject anxious thoughts that are habitual and recurring.

The key ingredient in self-reflection is detachment, a concept that grows deeper and deeper with each limb of Yoga. Here detachment doesn't imply indifference, passivity, or apathy. Instead, you distance yourself from the pull of emotion.

Let's say that you get word that someone you trust, such as a close friend, uttered a harsh criticism about you that has gotten back to you. A flush of anger rises in you. You may feel sad or angry and wonder why you ever thought this person was a real friend. Perhaps the temptation to exact revenge or to say damaging things about your friend enters the picture.

You have several opportunities to practice detachment here. First, at the instant anger starts to rise, you can pause, take a deep breath, and hold up your hand for time-out. Second, you can sit quietly until your immediate reaction dies down and reason can prevail. Perhaps your friend didn't actually say what was reported to you, or perhaps a slight has been blown out of all proportion. Third, you can close your eyes, center yourself, and do a simple breathing meditation until your anger dissipates. Finally, you can reflect on the fact that you have survived worse criticism and will seek a way to understand and forgive your friend.

What these four possibilities have in common is that you move closer to your true self, which is never wounded, cares nothing about criticism, sees everyone in the light of loving acceptance, and brings compassion and forgiveness to any situation. The opposite of self-reflection is to nurse your grievance against your friend, indulging in a combination of self-pity and fantasies of getting even. Learning a better way to respond emotionally is the whole purpose of the *niyamas*, and detachment is an important skill to be learned.

Exercise

Consider the example of an angry response given above. Reflect on how it applies to your own store of resentments, grudges, and old hurts from other people. Go inside and reflect on moving these emotional residues so that you bring a sense of light and lightness to your feelings. To make your ability to self-reflect even more powerful, be on the lookout the next time you have a strong impulse to be angry, envious, anxious, or discouraged. In the moment of your reaction, pause and follow the four opportunities mentioned in the anger example above. Genuinely try to adopt detachment as your response, looking upon it as a skill based on emotional intelligence. You can journal about how the experience allowed you to see how self-reflection and detachment work, and how much you can benefit from simply taking a step back and expanding your vision of who you really are.

FRIDAY

Surrender to the Unknown

Begin by silently repeating today's theme:

I give myself over to the great mystery.
I give myself over to the great mystery.

The fifth and final *niyama* asks you to recognize your higher reality and surrender to it. In daily life there is a constant push-pull between getting what you want and giving in to what someone else wants. Giving in is a form of surrender, which is why most people do not like the connotation of that word. It seems foreign to human nature when this *niyama* calls for complete surrender.

The issue hasn't been cleared up by Yoga commentaries that use a mix-and-match vocabulary, some calling for surrender to God, others making it surrender to the Absolute, the divine mystery of existence or Brahman (the Sanskrit word for "big" that implies the whole of creation, the One, the All).

To gain clarity, first we must sweep away all this loaded vocabulary. As a famous Yogic saying affirms, "Those who speak of It know It not. Those who know It speak of It not." Here *It* refers to God/the Absolute/the divine mystery/Brahman, according to the terminology you favor. Names don't matter, because the "real" reality is beyond language.

With this understanding in mind, the fifth *niyama* isn't about ordinary surrender, which involves giving in to someone else and thus sacrificing what you want. In Royal Yoga, surrender is simply the recognition of higher reality. Once accepted, there is an end to seeking, frustration, and endless speculation. Religious history is full of all three, so this isn't religious surrender, either. You acknowledge your place in the mystery of existence.

Then what? Once you accept that water is wet, there's not much more to say. The fifth *niyama* teaches that the contemplation of higher reality brings endless rewards. The practices of contemplation will make this clearer.

THE PRACTICES OF CONTEMPLATION

Welcome the end of seeking.

Turn your attention to what life means.

Expose yourself to inspirational poetry and scripture.

Attune yourself to the beauty of Nature.

Follow your creative impulses.

Act from your finest feelings whenever you can.

Take time to offer gratitude.

Dwell on your version of a higher being or consciousness.

Nurture awe and wonder in the contemplation of creation.

See yourself as having a unique place in the divine or cosmic plan.

These practices are meant to have a direct personal effect. The effect is to get you out of linear thinking—this isn't a journey from A to B, but a journey to show you who you have always been.

In that light, the practices of contemplation constantly expand our self-awareness. We are all used to expanding our awareness, even if we don't label it as such. As an example, consider when we learned to read. The state of literacy opens an entirely new way of being. When your contemplation practice opens up even a moment of insight, joy, or inspiration, this signals how total transformation will be. The process begins by surrendering to the reality that the source of creation exists and is identical to your source, the true self.

Exercise

In detective fiction, a mystery is something that needs solving, and, until it is solved, things haven't been set right. The guilty need to be unmasked; right must prevail. But the mystery of the source is different. The human mind exists in the relative world. But this doesn't present an impenetrable barrier to the Absolute—quite the opposite. To use a traditional image from Yoga, imagine that the Absolute is sending arrows of light into the created world.

Consider that the highest values in life, including love, compassion, creativity, empathy, beauty, truth, and spiritual inspiration, are what the arrows carry to our world. This is a good start for practicing contemplation. Sit quietly and let your mind go to an experience of one of those values just listed. Feel the lightness, vibrancy, joy, and fulfillment your experience contained. Let these subtle feelings expand and settle in your awareness. You are learning the truth of the Yogic saying "This isn't knowledge you learn. This is knowledge you become."

ADVANCED EXPLORATION

If you want to go more deeply into classic Yoga, there are many sources of information about the *niyamas*, beginning with all the free information online. Look under the Sanskrit names for the *niyamas*, which are given below with their traditional translations.

Saucha: Clean body, mind, and spirit
Santosha: Contentment
Tapas: Austerities, self-discipline
Svadhyaya: Self-reflection
Ishvara pranidhana: Surrender to or contemplation of a Supreme Being

BRINGING THE LIGHT TO YOUR BODY

(Limb of Yoga: *Asana*)

THIS PART OF THE JOURNEY

The third limb of Yoga, known as *asana*, is about making a conscious connection with your body. From there a union of equals—a spiritual marriage—can be experienced. Without this connection, there is no true knowledge of who you really are.

The term *asana* has been adopted for the postures that Sarah deals with in Part II of the book. Each posture is specifically aimed at changes in biology and physiology that affect your mood and mental state. A precise science underlies this branch of Yoga. It is an inner science, despite the physical image of a yogi sitting in lotus position that most people see when they think of Yoga.

In Week 3, I will focus on the inner science, presenting the pure view of Patanjali, which holds that the body is a disguised form of consciousness. Remove the disguise—cells, tissues, organs, and systems—and you will discover how to bring your body into the light. Perhaps it is fairer to say that your body is going to bring you into the light.

MONDAY

The Conscious Body

Begin by silently repeating today's theme:

I experience my body as a flow of awareness.
I experience my body as a flow of awareness.

Your body isn't a machine, even a miraculous machine, but a storehouse of infinite knowledge. If we look at any process in the body, from a cell dividing to reproduce itself to the immune system repelling an invader or the digestive tract extracting energy from food, a vast amount of knowledge is on display. No process is mechanical. The body's knowledge is alive, flowing, and conscious.

Royal Yoga aims to bring the body fully into the light. When you mistreat your body—subjecting your body to stress, bad diet, and poor-quality sleep—its consciousness is dulled. When you fail to tune into the signals your body sends to you, you are denying that it is conscious. These are *vrittis* that block the light. Until they are overcome, you won't fully experience freedom, joy, and bliss, because your body is the vehicle for all higher experiences.

At its most basic, *asana*, the Sanskrit word for "seat," teaches you to settle comfortably into your body as the seat, or foundation, that determines your place in the physical world. The body in motion is one thing, dynamic and changeable. The seat is another thing, unchanging, stable, and continuously present.

BRINGING THE LIGHT TO YOUR BODY

Realize that every cell is eavesdropping on your thoughts, feelings, and sensations.

See your body as your willing ally.

Drop the habit of blaming or disparaging your body.

Don't compare your body to an unreachable ideal.

Obey your body's signals, particularly its need for sleep and the regulation of stress.

Avoid prolonged sessions of sitting down—move and stretch for a few minutes every hour.

Look upon your body as new every day.

Make lifelong wellness your goal.

Bringing light and lightness to your body comes naturally once you see your body as being aware and knowing. The life that flows through every cell is vibrant. Your role is to let your whole body express this vibrancy. There are physical, mental, and psychological ways to accomplish this, but everything begins with acknowledging the conscious body as your default attitude.

Exercise

Sit quietly with your eyes closed and take a few deep breaths. When you feel calm and centered, visualize an outline of your body. Keeping the outline in mind, start filling it in with light. An easy way to do this is to see light expanding from the center of the image, the heart, and radiating outward as a soft white glow. Another aid is to feel yourself breathing the light into the outline.

Continue for 5 to 10 minutes, then relax with your eyes closed. Move easily back into your daily activity. Notice if you feel more light and lightness physically, which is the goal of this exercise. Don't be concerned if you don't. Your awareness has lightened your body all the same, and if you keep this practice up, the experience of lightness will appear and grow stronger.

TUESDAY

Presence

Begin by silently repeating today's theme:

I join my body in the present moment.
I join my body in the present moment.

Do you think you are living in the present moment? The concept of the "power of now" has been widely popularized, and so have practices for living in the present. Yoga looks upon this issue differently. There is no power in the present moment when you adopt the viewpoint of the timeless. A moment is a mind-made construct. What matters is presence, which is timeless. Presence comes from the light. Without attaching the word *divine* to it, presence is felt as a combination of alertness and openness that makes the now feel perfect just by being here.

Without presence, the now is a blank. The pathos of the elderly when dementia strikes is that they are present the way a chair or a rock is present, as a passive, inert body in which awareness barely flickers. The infinite field of pure awareness is the source of presence; therefore, being fully present is your natural state—babies are fully present, as you can see by the look of wonder and curiosity in their eyes.

As it was designed, your body is an unfailing guide for living in the present moment, because that's where every cell lives—it never loses sight of the now. Asana points to the *vidya*, or "wisdom of the body," as a given, yet this wisdom gets distorted and contradicted by the activity of the mind. The effect of this distortion is easy to see.

THE WISDOM OF THE BODY

Every cell in the body knows how to live in peace with every other cell. It is the mind that has invented violence.

Cells exist to keep the whole body alive. The mind has invented selfishness and separation.

Cells communicate freely. The mind keeps secrets.

Cells trust in a stream of food and oxygen that is constantly renewed. The mind has invented mistrust.

Cells are born and die without fear. The mind dreads death.

The body maintains itself in perfect dynamic balance. The mind is driven toward bursts of manic activity and paralyzed depression.

The body heals itself automatically. The mind struggles to heal itself.

Absent the *vrittis*, the body lives fully in the here and now, aware of everything it needs to know. Which of us can say the same thing? The upshot is that the mind needs to be deposed as the be-all and end-all of human awareness. For most people, no matter how much they blame or criticize their bodies, it is the body that is ahead in their evolution, not the mind.

Exercise

Get in the habit of respecting your body's wisdom by listening to what it is telling you. Take time to sit with your eyes closed and simply feel your body. Let your attention go wherever it wants to. If you sense discomfort, tightness, stiffness, stress, or painful sensations, let your awareness rest there. Take deep breaths, relax, and notice if the sensation begins to lessen. Feeling the body is healing the body. We don't realize this truth because we are in the habit of withdrawing our awareness from signals of physical discomfort, stress, or pain.

One reason that the healing response works while we are asleep is that the body is allowed to bring full awareness to the process. Once we wake up, we tend to diminish the healing response by forcing our awareness elsewhere. In essence, we deny the healing response an open field in which to work. Much of this opposition happens unconsciously, and feeling the body is a gentle exercise for replacing your unconscious reaction with a conscious response instead.

WEDNESDAY

Staying Grounded

Begin by silently repeating today's theme:

I rest comfortably in my body.
I rest comfortably in my body.

If animals could talk, we don't know what they'd say, but we can be certain about what they wouldn't say: "I hate my body." Hating your body is a uniquely human response and an unnatural one. Royal Yoga holds that a healthy relationship with your body begins by being comfortable with your physicality. The modern term for this is being *grounded*. We say that a person is grounded if they are sensible, realistic, reliable, and not given to flights of fancy. Those are good traits, but asana is about being grounded in yourself, which occurs only as your awareness deepens.

It is peculiar to stand back and discover just how much judgment has been leveled against physicality itself, which the body symbolizes. Long-held religious beliefs denigrate the physical for pulling us down from the heights of the spiritual. Physicality reminds us of our low, knuckle-dragging primate forebears. To be physical is to be brutish; to be spiritual is divine.

Yet as Yoga sees it, one flow of consciousness supports life in every dimension. There is no reason to denigrate the physical once you realize how much wisdom (*vidya*) is expressed in every cell, the wisdom of life as a whole. Yoga takes us beyond the deceptive look of the body—solid, material, fixed in time and space—to the reality. We aren't embodied in a body; we are embodied in awareness.

What follows are the qualities that represent being fully grounded.

YOU ARE GROUNDED WHEN...
Being embodied brings you joy.
You understand the deep wisdom of your body.
You feel attuned to Nature.
You cherish the Earth for creating earthly existence.
You feel unembarrassed by basic bodily functions.
You appreciate other people's earthiness.
You feel stable and steady during periods of change.
You experience equanimity in the face of aging and dying.
Your sensual and sexual life is gratifying, without prudery or shame.

When you watch little children romping in the mud or running around the house unencumbered, how does your response reflect on you? What we call the innocence of childhood exists, yes, but it is more appropriately called being grounded. Children feel no impulse, unless they are mistreated, to be disembodied. They have no need to renounce or escape their physical nature.

This naturally grounded state changes as soon as the mind intervenes to create certain attitudes that drive us to become disembodied—not like ghosts but as creatures who judge against our physicality.

YOU BECOME DISEMBODIED WHEN . . .

You don't feel comfortable inside your own skin.

Your body arouses in you distaste or disgust.

You remember physical experiences that led to humiliation, guilt, or shame.

You live in your head.

You always choose indoor distractions over going out into Nature.

You hold negative views of the human body. These may be religious (seeing the body as sinful) or based on personal aversion (for example, being repelled by the body's messier functions).

Physical beauty or ugliness becomes a fixation.

You have poor body image because you are overweight, aging, or subject to social attitudes about physical perfection and desirability.

You don't feel physically lovable or desirable.

You neglect to keep your body clean, well cared for, and active.

You think that earthy people are stupid or crude.

When we list all the ways we put down our bodies, it becomes evident that we live in a disembodied age to a shocking degree. Mass media overloads us with fantasies of a perfect body that never ages while robbing us of the real blessing of being embodied. The embodied state allows us to feel the physical side of bliss-consciousness, which is a vibrant sense of aliveness as we move through our day.

Exercise

Every step you take to welcome your own physicality is a step into the light. Look at the two lists above that outline the qualities of being grounded versus the qualities of being disembodied. Pause to reflect on how you can adopt more grounded beliefs and turn them into enjoyable actions, like walking in Nature, participating in a sport, taking part in forms of physical recreation, or going for a massage.

As you engage in this activity, no matter how simple it is—you might just lie spread-eagle on the warm ground in summer or (believe it or not) hug a tree—reflect on how blessed you are to be embodied. Bring a positive feeling toward your body whenever you can. Drop the casual habit of disparaging your body. Through these steady steps of becoming more grounded, you are removing another layer of obstacles between you and your true self.

THURSDAY

Resilience

Begin by silently repeating today's theme:

I bend flexibly with every experience.
I bend flexibly with every experience.

The physical flexibility that comes from practicing the asanas, or postures of yoga, is visible evidence of something rooted in consciousness: resilience. Bad things happen to everyone, no matter how much we wish they wouldn't. What matters is not the bad things themselves but how we respond after they occur. Resilience is the ability to bounce back from pain and adversity. The opposite of resilience is being stuck and unable to move on.

Listing the qualities of resilience erases the line we draw between physical, mental, and psychological. It requires a holistic conception to really embrace your own resilience, which can take you beyond surviving to thriving in the face of changing experiences.

YOU SHOW RESILIENCE WHEN ...

You bend and adapt to change.

Your body is flexible and agile.

You are open-minded toward people who are different from you.

You don't exaggerate what happened in the past.

You let your emotions rise and fall naturally, without trying to force or suppress them.

You don't insist on always being right.

You are not afraid of what life brings you.

The future holds no apprehension.

The emotional state of others doesn't throw you.

You can renounce the belief "My way is best."

You face new challenges with optimism.

You view every day as a new world.

You stretch yourself in any way you define that term.

None of these qualities is meant to be forced. They are a natural part of everyone's existence. It takes effort to move away from resilience into the condition of rigidity, or stuckness. It isn't necessary to go into detail about all the ways that stuckness occurs. We all have a good grasp of what is involved, but if you need a reminder, return to the list above and just flip each entry to its opposite. If you don't adapt to change, don't approach challenges optimistically, don't accept people who are different from you, and so on through the list, you are rigid and stuck.

Why do we stay stuck? We get a false sense of security from being rigid in our ways. We put up an inflexible front to the world, yet behind it, we are afraid to be truly open, free, accepting, emotionally honest, and optimistic. In a state of fear, something as precious as love becomes a source of anxiety if we have experienced enough unloving behavior and been scarred by it.

Learning to be resilient should proceed with an eye to your inner comfort and discomfort. A stiff emotional body needs to be treated with care, like a stiff physical body. The important thing is to resist the false security of being rigid and stuck—the shell you are hiding inside is suffocating to the spirit.

Exercise

Having read this discussion, no doubt you can see where you are resilient and where you are stuck. There is always a path to follow that shifts the balance, day by day, toward becoming more resilient. To stay on the path, however, it must be appealing and bring satisfaction. Besides bringing a false sense of security, being stuck makes you feel good, after a fashion, because you know that you are always right, that you don't need to change, and that your fixed beliefs and attitudes are fine just the way they are.

The key warning here is that your stuckness indulges an illusion. Giving up on love, for example, indulges a person's anxiety about asking for and receiving love. Somehow you need to break the ice that makes being stuck cold and lonely, no matter how good the front you put up. Start by looking over the listed qualities of resilience and, for each one, devise a step you can take that will feel good enough for you to continue on the path.

You might stand and stretch while listening to music, moving on to dance exercises you can do at home. You might spend more time with the happiest people you know or show a little more affection to a family member than either of you expect. Resilience isn't a trait society teaches us to value, but that doesn't matter. Awareness, like pure water, needs to flow, and being resilient is how you open the gates inside yourself.

FRIDAY

In Perfect Sync

Begin by silently repeating today's theme:

I live in the flow of creative intelligence.
I live in the flow of creative intelligence.

You are designed to have mind and body in perfect sync. One of the greatest deceptions in life is the helpless appearance presented by a newborn baby. Unable to do much more than nurse at the breast, cry, and sleep, a day-old infant doesn't reveal what it really is—a miracle of organized intelligence. In the last few days of pregnancy, for example, the infant brain is developing millions of new brain cells a day. This process continues after the infant is born. It is beyond imagination how a brain that has no language, reason, fully formed emotions, or ideas prepared itself for all of that, and more. It's as if a house knew how to build itself from the materials in the aisles of Home Depot.

Self-creation cannot happen on the physical plane without consciousness. You can't assemble the ingredients of a neuron and expect it to reach a tipping point when—*Voila!*—a swirl of chemical soup becomes conscious.

If existence were ideal, mind and body would remain in perfect synchronization, and in a healthy person they work flawlessly 99 percent of the time. It takes interference to throw off the flow of creative intelligence that unites mind and body. The symptoms of meddling are all too common.

SYMPTOMS OF BEING OUT OF SYNC

Irregular or poor-quality sleep, insomnia

Fatigue, lack of energy

Depression

Digestive problems

Overeating, loss of natural hunger rhythms

Inability to focus and pay attention

Susceptibility to colds and infections

Getting easily distracted

Sensitivity to minor stress

Slow or inadequate healing

This whole list could be titled "When the miracle goes wrong." Each of these symptoms indicates that the miraculous flow of creative intelligence that everyone was gifted with at birth has become distorted. Without the word *creative* added, the picture is woefully incomplete. Once it has been programmed, a computer can imitate intelligence by doing all kinds of things the mind does, and AI (artificial intelligence) is fast reaching the day when the imitation will be so lifelike that your computer will sound and feel human. Already there are software programs that effectively conduct psychotherapy, for example. A robot voice imitates a genuine therapist using verbal prompts like "How do you feel about that?" and "When did you start to feel this way?" Users of the program come away feeling better, they say.

But no matter how sophisticated AI becomes, it cannot do what you do every second: take raw information pouring into the brain from the five senses and create the entire three-dimensional world you perceive. Cameras aren't eyes. They see nothing. Therefore, a computer camera sees nothing until a human eye is present. When you were in the womb, creative intelligence created your eye from a blob of undifferentiated cells, and within the eye specific cells were assigned to carry out visual processing. Yet that isn't enough for turning visual images into something you see. Vision happens in the perfect interface between mind and the visual cortex of the brain.

Royal Yoga teaches you how to keep the flow of creative intelligence from being distorted and blocked. If you fall out of sync, exhibiting the symptoms listed above, you must get out of the way and allow creative intelligence to restore what has gone awry. The practices aren't new or surprising. It's a matter of doing what we already know as right living.

GETTING BACK IN SYNC

Practice grounding and rest comfortably in yourself.

Take care to get 8 to 9 hours of sound sleep every night, preferably uninterrupted.

Establish regular hours for eating and sleeping.

Avoid physical and mental exhaustion.

Keep mentally active.

Don't put toxins in your body. Don't put toxic experiences in your mind.

Take time to center yourself if you feel distracted, stressed, upset, or overwhelmed.

Meditate every day, using any method you choose—taking the time is more important than the technique.

Go out into Nature and let the experience bring deep relaxation.

Take your own well-being as seriously as you take work, family, and relationships.

Learn a physical skill that requires mind-body coordination (yoga, dancing, aerobics, sports, physical recreation, etc.).

You might look upon this list as familiar advice, but every piece forms part of the mystery of existence. Everything that went into the evolution of Homo sapiens was the result of being in perfect sync with creative intelligence.

Creative intelligence has an intention in mind for you personally, not simply for our species. Being in perfect sync isn't like making sure to tune up your car to keep it in top running order. Being in perfect sync is about your evolution, and your evolution is about reaching your source so that you can live in the light.

Exercise

If you look over the two lists that describe the opposite conditions of being in or out of sync, a spark of recognition will grow inside you. This spark indicates that more light and lightness comes from being in sync than from being out of sync. The unblocked flow of creative intelligence makes your existence more vibrant, alert, receptive, avid, buoyant, and appreciative. Take up an activity that brings those qualities to life. Don't settle for the passive state of inertia. Even simple physical activity that makes you feel more alert and alive is evolutionary. Evolution is the whole game, and you are evolving when an experience makes you feel new and renewed. The same desire drives every cell in your body, so it is only natural for you to share in it fully and perfectly.

VITAL ENERGY

(Limb of Yoga: *Pranayama*)

THIS PART OF THE JOURNEY

Every limb of Royal Yoga reveals what is required to lead an ideal life. The fourth limb, known as *pranayama*, is concerned with the free flow of the life force or vital energy known as prana. In the Yoga system, the flow of prana is life-giving, but unlike physical energy, prana is conscious. Therefore, it responds to our state of consciousness.

This is of critical importance. The experience of being alive here and now is meant to be vital and vibrant. Mind and body are alert, and the energy we associate with youth is present for a lifetime. Ideally, Royal Yoga provides a pathway to lifelong energy and vitality.

Yet this is one area where the gap between an ideal life and real life is very wide. Time is a falling arc. We expect to age, and although the "new old age" has raised our expectations in terms of overall health and life expectancy, the gap remains.

This brings up a fact that most people aren't aware of: Aging is a mysterious process that no one has adequately defined. No two people age in the same way. At the moment of death, the cause is typically the breakdown of a single organ or system. If life is based on DNA, which is a strand of simple organic chemicals, then we should be protected from the rigors of old age, because our basic chemical components—carbon, oxygen, hydrogen, and nitrogen—don't age. Most of the atoms in your body are as ancient as stars.

A single explanation for aging seems impossible and yet is the very thing we need. Royal Yoga offers a very simple explanation: We age when prana, the life force, declines. Like atoms and molecules, prana itself doesn't age, but it can weaken in a person over time. The fourth limb of Yoga is devoted to practices of breath control—in Sanskrit *prana* means "breath." Traditionally, there are dozens of breathing exercises that aim to direct the breath for very specific purposes in the body, including the prevention of aging.

This week we will touch upon breathing from a different angle. Prana, once you go deeply into it, is about the meeting point between every atom in creation and the spark of life that animates not just our bodies, but the cosmos.

MONDAY

Breath of Life

Begin by silently repeating today's theme:

I join the flow of life with every breath.
I join the flow of life with every breath.

Nature designed us to breathe through our nose, a fact we never bother to notice until the onset of a cold, allergies, or another condition that obstructs nasal breathing. It seems amazing, therefore, that Yoga hit upon the discovery that breathing through your nose has a hidden purpose—it is the portal through which prana enters the body.

By controlling your breath at the portal, you can potentially direct prana anywhere at will. Yoga provides a road map of the subtle pathways (or *nadis*) that prana follows. The map looks very much like the network of blood vessels and nerves mapped by modern medical anatomy. Yoga teaches that vital energy is always moving. You are most alive when you feel vibrant with energy; someone is sick or in decline when they are drained of energy. But, at a deeper level, prana follows the path laid out by consciousness, which is the true creative force in you and every living creature.

Since the *nadis* are invisible channels and prana can't be measured objectively, it doesn't have a place in modern medicine. Only by exploring their own consciousness did the ancient Vedic *rishis*, or seers, discover it in the first place. In practical terms, Royal Yoga is concerned with how the free flow of prana can increase your quality of life. Its benefits are experienced personally, beginning with the mind, which makes sense since prana is the conduit, or carrier, of consciousness.

PRANA IS FLOWING FREELY WHEN . . .

Your mind is alert, and you are thinking clearly.

You feel peaceful inside.

A quiet mind is accompanied by easy, regular breathing.

The mental *vrittis* of anxiety, worry, and anger settle down and eventually vanish.

You experience a natural feeling of well-being.

Your mental state is unaffected by stress.

You have a sense of freshness that renews itself every day.

Immediately you can see that the state of prana determines the quality of a person's life. You are designed, according to Yoga, so that prana is flowing freely when you are simply breathing through your nose. Mouth breathing is associated with imbalanced states in the body. Any imbalance serves as a ready indicator of blocked or decreased prana. Leaving aside colds, allergies, and medical conditions that block breathing, people mouth-breathe when they are anxious, stressed, exhausted, or depressed, or when they suffer from insomnia or sleep apnea. All these disturbed conditions are also associated with decreased energy, both physical and mental.

PRANA IS BLOCKED WHEN...

You feel fatigued or exhausted.

You lose mental clarity.

You experience anxiety.

You display nervousness.

You lose a sense of inner calm.

You can't pay attention without being easily distracted.

Your have muscle weakness and lose muscle tone.

You show signs of aging.

You become prone to colds, flu, and random infections.

You heal more slowly than normal.

Mouth breathing is medically connected with sleep apnea. More intriguing is how complex the human nose is when examined, not for the sense of smell, but for what happens as air enters. The tiny fibers that line the nasal passage are remarkably effective at filtering out airborne particles (up to 20 billion a day, according to one estimate) as well as warming the air being inhaled in cold weather and cooling it in warm weather, enhancing the smooth operation of the lungs. There is also a moistening effect in the nose's mucous membranes that is beneficial to the lungs.

Yet Royal Yoga is more focused on how prana functions as the breath of life, meaning that it transmits the living energy that knows how the body—indeed, all of creation—should be knit together as a single living organism. From the cell to the cosmos, the flow of prana is synonymous with the flow of creative intelligence.

Exercise

On its own, breathing through your nose naturally allows prana to flow freely. A simple breath meditation like the following is recommended for everyone. You can adopt it as a daily practice or turn to it anytime during your day when you want to be calmer, more centered, and quieter inside.

Sitting in a quiet place with low lighting, close your eyes and take a few deep breaths until you feel settled and ready to meditate. Don't shorten or skip these introductory moments. They prepare your breathing to get in sync with your state of awareness.

Direct your attention to the tip of your nose and sense air as it passes in and out with each breath. (After a moment, if you feel that your breathing is short, ragged, irregular, or gasping, take time to lie down without meditating and let your breathing return to normal.) Continue to easily follow the in-and-out rhythm of your breathing. Don't force a rhythm, and don't mind if you occasionally draw a deep sigh or feel that you must take a breath through your mouth. These are good signs, since they indicate that your breathing is working to rebalance itself.

Continue doing this for 5 to 20 minutes. If you notice your attention wandering, just gently bring it back to the tip of your nose. When time is up, lie down or sit quietly to let yourself return from the meditative state.

Don't rush back into activity. Take as much time as you need to readjust to a relaxed waking state, ready for your next activity.

TUESDAY

The Key to Stronger Breathing

Begin by silently repeating today's theme:

My breathing energizes mind and body.
My breathing energizes mind and body.

When your breathing is strong, so is your prana. Every function in the body is improved by having an optimal level of oxygen in the blood, but aging, respiratory problems, allergies, and air pollution bring most people down from this optimal level. Breath, in a way, is like the old adage "For want of a nail, the kingdom was lost"—incremental changes in breathing can trigger a decline by small degrees in critical areas like blood pressure, heart health, and brain function. The upshot is that almost everyone can benefit by strengthening their breathing so that small deficits don't take hold.

We aren't dealing in this book with traditional controlled Yogic breathing, which requires a teacher and a committed discipline, but conscious breathing is something everyone can and should learn. Breath is the portal of prana, and conscious breathing practices rank high for improving the flow of prana.

Here are three breathing exercises that have been well researched and validated.

#1 Belly Breathing

This exercise is based on the understanding that the lower area of the lungs stimulates relaxation. Shallow breathing, which mostly uses the upper part of the lungs, is associated with stress, anxiety, and panic attacks. The aim of belly breathing is to use your diaphragm as you consciously take in a full, deep breath.

Sit upright and start to breathe slowly. With each in-breath, feel the air going to the bottom of your abdomen as you swell your belly out. Move your diaphragm outward, making sure that you breathe slowly, and don't strain. When your belly feels full, breathe out by letting your lungs expel the air naturally, the way you would let go of a sigh.

Repeat for 5 to 10 minutes, always breathing through your nose. If you feel the impulse to breathe through your mouth or to gasp, don't resist. Try not to push yourself. Like all breathing exercises, this one should feel comfortable. In time, you will build up more endurance.

#2 Vagal Breathing

The vagus nerve, which is one of the ten cranial nerves leading directly from the brain, has received a great deal of publicity in recent years. The vagus nerve plays a major role in regulating heartbeat, breathing, and the intestines; it tells your body whether you are stressed—all three organs are involved in triggering the fight-or-flight response.

By gently stimulating the vagus nerve, you send signals of relaxation and the absence of stress throughout your body. Vagal breathing is the simplest way to stimulate the vagus nerve, yet it turns out to be one of the most effective ways to counter low-level chronic stress, which almost everyone in modern life is subjected to.

Sit quietly, breathing through your nose. Slowly and comfortably draw in a breath, making sure it is deep enough to fill your lungs. Hold for a few seconds, then slowly release your breath. The essential thing here is to consciously draw in a breath, pausing without strain, and consciously exhaling. The awareness of breathing is just as important as the technique being used.

Repeat for 5 to 10 minutes. Vagal breathing is thought to have many more benefits than relaxing and diminishing the stress response, but those benefits on their own make it valuable.

Vagal breathing will be effective for some people, but if you find that slow, conscious breathing only increases the impulse to breathe in a shallow, ragged way (which is typical in situations of acute stress) or if you feel the slightest signs of panic, discontinue this practice. In such situations, lying down and breathing normally with the eyes closed will start to bring the body out of the stress response. This can be followed up by meditating, but, again, if going inward makes you overly aware of your stress and anxiety, stop meditating and sit quietly, being gently aware of your body and your breath.

#3 Regulated Breathing

This is an advanced exercise, since it is related to formal techniques of *pranayama*. Yet regulated breathing is a natural step from vagal breathing. In this exercise, you are asked to count your breaths, bringing conscious control to the act of breathing.

Sit quietly, breathing through your nose. If you feel a little distracted or tense, take a few deep breaths until you feel relaxed and settled. Now breathe in slowly to the count of 4, exhale slowly to the count of 8, then count to 8 before taking your next breath; in other words 4-8-8 for one breath cycle. Even at this early stage, regulated breathing can be a little challenging for some, since it runs counter to the habit of unconscious breathing that everyone is used to.

But the practice is worth mastering, because it brings about deep relaxation and changes in brain-wave activity. Simply by regulating your breath, you can go into the meditative state represented by increased alpha-wave activity. With practice, it is possible to put the brain into the same state as deep sleep while still remaining alert and awake.

If this prospect intrigues you, first become comfortable over a period of days with a 4-8-8 rhythm. Then move on to longer periods. Your goal is 6-12-12; in other words, inhaling to a count of 6, exhaling to a count of 12, then waiting for a count of 12 before taking your next breath.

One effect of regulated breathing is to slow down the number of breaths you take per minute. The average number for someone at rest is 12 to 16 breaths per minute. Regulated breathing slows the rate down drastically, and if you attain a count of 6-12-12, you may be breathing as little as two times per minute. Advanced yogis can slow their breathing (along with heartbeat and oxygen consumption) to a level that reaches the state of consciousness closest to the source (*samadhi*).

An intriguing possibility is held out for people in their everyday lives. Yoga measures a lifetime not by years but by how many breaths are taken. Slower breathing, if done consciously, involves few breaths per minute, resulting in a longer life span. The general concept makes sense. Breathing slowly indicates a relaxed state that is less affected by stress. How long someone's life span can be extended is open to further research, but the benefits of a calmer mind, deeper awareness, and better regulated physiology are beyond doubt.

WEDNESDAY

Prana and the Light

Begin by silently repeating today's theme:

I direct all my energies to the light
I direct all my energies to the light.

When we talk about improving the quality of life, what we should say is the *qualities* of life. An ideal life is built upon them. By comparison, if you focus on externals, like money, status, and possessions, as markers of the good life, you haven't even touched the qualities that matter. As prana circulates through your body, it animates every cell with the primary qualities that also bring vital energy to you as a person.

THE PRIMARY QUALITIES OF PRANA

Freshness, renewal
Vitality, vibrancy
Creativity
Self-sufficiency
Intelligence
Growth, evolution

These are the qualities that make prana a living energy, and they give us a direct connection to the light, because prana is the carrier of consciousness. Yoga holds that consciousness is more powerful the closer you get to the source. Prana circulates at a subtle level that is much closer to the source than the physical processes of the body.

Every breath brings in life-giving oxygen, which has chemical properties that interact with the physical properties of thousands of other molecules at the cellular level. But the cell would have no life without the
qualities listed above. Think of scrap iron rusting in a junkyard. Two atoms
of oxygen and iron are involved, and the net result is that the iron gets
broken down and deteriorates.

The same oxygen and iron atoms interact in your bloodstream, impart-
ing the color to red blood corpuscles. Yet the effect is the exact opposite of
rusted iron. The oxygen is used to nourish the qualities of life—refreshing
every cell, giving it vitality, allowing the cell to sustain itself and grow.
Without the qualities of life carried by prana, the physical side of life would
deteriorate into random chemical reactions, leading to chaos and decay.

Prana automatically tends to the qualities of life as you breathe, but you
can choose to expand or diminish its effectiveness. What gives you control
over prana is your state of awareness. Since prana has the same source in
pure awareness that you do, it is affected by your mental state. Consider
two psychological states—anxiety and depression—that hamper the flow of
prana. When prana is weakened, life feels dull, enervated, insecure, exhausting, overwhelming in its daily functioning, and without any sense of
vibrancy. These are precisely the clinical description of depression and anxiety.

The drugs used to treat anxiety and depression do not actually cure
those conditions. This failing has always been a thorn in the side for psy-
chiatry, but Royal Yoga points to a much more significant phenomenon.
The same areas of the brain affected by these drugs are similarly affected
through talk, or couch, therapy. In other words, exchanging words with a
therapist about how you feel—the qualities of life as you experience them—

can alleviate anxiety and depression as effectively as drugs and with no side effects. Yoga's explanation for this is that going to the level of qualities (i.e., subjective experience) allows prana to be consciously redirected back into a healthier pattern.

This is a prime example of the basic insight Royal Yoga delivers: You can only change what you are aware of. Awareness guides prana, and prana communicates to your cells the changes you want to make.

Exercise

The basic takeaway today is that changing the quality of your life depends on changing the many qualities of your life. A blanket intention ("I want things to get better") isn't effective. What's effective is to focus on the primary qualities that prana carries as it moves through mind and body. Look at the list of qualities and begin to focus at first on one or two of them.

How can you make your life feel refreshed instead of routine? What creative activity can you take up? Which daily problems and challenges can you deal with more intelligently? Be specific. Write down the thoughts that come to you. A great help is to consult a trusted friend or family member who exemplifies the quality you want to develop. This can be someone who is strikingly creative or self-sufficient or smart about dealing with their own issues. When you engage in a stimulating back-and-forth, you are enlivening the flow of prana then and there, which is half the answer.

THURSDAY

Energy Healing

Begin by silently repeating today's theme:

I redirect my energy wherever it is needed.
I redirect my energy wherever it is needed.

Awareness brings change. Wherever you direct your awareness, a change occurs in the way prana flows. This principle lies at the heart of energy work, a broad term that can apply to traditional Eastern therapies, like Ayurveda, qi gong, and acupuncture, or to modern chiropractic and osteopathy. They all depend on redirecting vital energy at a subtle level.

Right at this moment, you are redirecting prana in ways that help to either promote or interfere with the healing process. You cannot change the pathways that prana flows through—these are as fixed as blood vessels or the central nervous system. But you can improve prana in several ways.

THE PRACTICES TO MAXIMIZE PRANA
Meditation
Controlling your breathing
Eating food that is as fresh as possible, drinking pure water, breathing pure, unpolluted air
Sleeping restfully and soundly
Reducing stress
Maintaining an optimistic outlook
Engaging in regular stretching and moving throughout the day

Going out into Nature
Avoiding mental and physical exhaustion

Nothing on this list is new or surprising, which is as it should be. Each limb of Yoga takes a different angle on the same goal, which is to achieve an ideal life. But constant reminders to do what is good for you aren't effective as motivation. You need to experience change in a healing direction, which then increases your desire for more of the same. In modern terminology, you need to create a positive feedback loop.

The simplest and most natural way to do that, when it comes to prana, is to get it moving. Flowing water remains fresh; stagnant water doesn't. The same holds true for prana. If you return to the list above, each practice spurs prana to circulate naturally, without exhausting or depleting your energy. Meditation might seem to be the exception, but it isn't. By calming the activity of the mind (*vrittis*), meditation opens the subtle channels through which prana flows.

Exercise

You can easily and gently bolster your prana by making your daily routine a little more conscious. Move and stretch every hour. Choose the freshest greens and vegetables in the market. Don't eat leftovers. Pay more attention to getting regular, good-quality sleep. Meditate, if only for a few minutes. These gradual changes require you to pay attention, and once a positive feedback loop is set up, it becomes more and more automatic. The watchwords with prana are *natural, unforced,* and *easy*—literally as easy as breathing.

FRIDAY

Eternal Creation

Begin by silently repeating today's theme:

I am part of a living, breathing creation.
I am part of a living, breathing creation.

Prana solves a mystery that otherwise defies explanation. If you look at a bumblebee from the perspective of an airplane engineer, the creature is too heavy, slow, and fat to fly. In a similar way, the human body shouldn't be alive if you look at it merely from a physical perspective. None of its chemical components are alive. If you take a quivering muscle cell or a pulsating heart cell and trace its makeup backward, from cell to molecules to atoms, the instant you take the first step, which brings you to the essential proteins that make up every cell, life has vanished. The most complex molecule inside you, your DNA, somehow learned the trick of dividing itself perfectly down the middle, and there's no doubt that life is based on passing on this trick so that cells can divide.

Ever since you started out as a single cell in your mother's womb, you have been the fortunate result of this trick. But DNA unzipping itself down the middle is still a purely chemical process, not all that distant from the way crystals multiply. Take a dense solution of sugar and water, suspend a string in it that has a single sugar crystal on it, and overnight many more crystals will magically surround it. A clump of sugar develops spontaneously and keeps on developing as long as the sugar solution is dense enough. But crystals aren't alive, and even when given billions of years to evolve, they never come to life.

The mystery of life disappears once you realize that everything is alive, and what keeps everything alive is prana. The spark of life isn't physical. Life is part of existence itself. It emerges at every level of creation, including the physical cosmos and the atom. Without creative intelligence, your body wouldn't survive another minute. At every level prana knows how to sustain life.

THE LIFE-GIVING FUNCTIONS OF PRANA
It brings nourishment to every cell.
It determines whether to create, destroy, or maintain life.
It promotes growth and evolution.
It organizes and regulates every process.
It synchronizes every biorhythm in the body.
It dynamically connects mind and body.

None of these functions can be explained through physical processes alone. Wherever creative intelligence flows, prana is flowing inside it. Physics employs matter and energy as the building blocks of creation, but this leaves out the critical element of intelligence.

Prana *knows* what it is doing. You can see how vitally important this is if you think of the electricity powering the lighting, heating, and appliances in your house. Can you conceive of the electrical current knowing the difference between a dryer, a fluorescent light, and a space heater before it reaches those appliances?

Yoga holds that everything in creation is a transformation of consciousness in different stages. The eight limbs of Yoga are levels of transformation. You can choose to expand your control over one level separately, the way *pranayama* controls breathing and asana controls physiology, but each limb is a facet of the whole. As a Vedic adage says, "Yoga is like a table with eight legs. Move one leg, and the whole table moves."

Pure consciousness is timeless, so is prana. The act of creation happening in your body in the next split second, which comprises hundreds of thousands of chemical reactions in a single cell, is the same act of creation that took place at the Big Bang and every moment afterward. So prana links you to eternal creation. Genesis, as Yoga sees it, is now.

Exercise

In your mind's eye, see yourself plucking an apple from a tree. Take a bite of the apple and swallow it. Mentally follow the path of the apple as it gets digested and gives up its energy. See the energy entering a heart cell and fueling a single heartbeat. Now ask yourself: At what point did life leave the apple? There were only stages of transformation as the fruit went from the tree to your heart. At each stage, different processes took over. (We could extend this example to the waste from the digested apple returning to the earth to nourish a seedling apple tree, perpetuating the circle of life.) Yet the chain of energy is unbroken, and so is the flow of life.

In this exercise you have grasped the eternal nature of prana. It moves, it morphs, it is guided from step to step by knowing what it needs to do. The link between life and consciousness is never broken, thanks to the vehicle that carries both life and consciousness, which is prana.

STAYING IN THE LIGHT

(Limb of Yoga: *Pratyahara*)

THIS PART OF THE JOURNEY

Royal Yoga is a journey to reach the ideal life. The fifth limb, known as *pratyahara*, is the turning point in this journey. Here you learn how to live in the light permanently. Instead of having a glimpse of love, compassion, creativity, beauty, truth, and the other values of higher consciousness, they are now your natural impulses. You get to experience them without the constantly churning mind blocking the way.

In classic Yoga, *pratyahara* is described as "the withdrawal of the senses," which isn't easy to grasp at first. If you are looking at an object—an apple, a television, another person—how can you not see it? Can you really withdraw your sense of sight? Yes, and you do it all the time by tuning out. You stop paying attention to what your eyes report and pay attention instead to your inner world. You can also hear without listening, which is why we say, "Sorry, I was distracted and didn't catch what you said." Your ears reported the sound of someone else talking, but your attention was elsewhere.

Once you tune out, *pratyahara* teaches you what to do next: Find the light and stay there. You know that you have accomplished this feat because the following things happen:

You experience your body as the gateway to bliss.
You melt away karmic impressions.
You conquer fear.
You see the evolutionary path and take it.
You start living from the level of solutions, instead of the level of
    problems.

In Week 5 we will cover the practices that lead to each of these victories, because that's what they are. The root causes of pain and suffering are defeated once and for all.

MONDAY

At Home in the Light

Begin by silently repeating today's theme:

I welcome the light as it welcomes me.
I welcome the light as it welcomes me.

The light is where you belong. This is one of the most basic truths revealed by Royal Yoga. Where you belong can also be called "home," so whatever home feels like, living in the light should feel the same way. The qualities of home are known to everyone. A child growing up in a secure, loving family learns what home represents, and these impressions last a lifetime. Home is, or should be:

Welcoming

Familiar

Safe

Relaxing

Happy

Loving

Nurturing

A child fortunate enough to experience these things simply by coming home depends on the parents to create these qualities. In Royal Yoga, you discover that they exist in yourself—the light provides them. The fifth limb of Yoga, *pratyahara*, teaches you how to settle down in the light, look around, and know what home really is. It's the place where you can be yourself. Ordinarily, you leave home to go out into the world and come back again, over and over, throughout your lifetime. In *pratyahara*, making the light your home is different because you can remain there without ever leaving.

Discovering that this is possible represents a breakthrough. Previously, the first four limbs of Yoga involved coming and going. You are navigating constant changes in the world around you, in your experiences, and in the activity of mind and body. *Pratyahara* merges coming and going by degrees until you become like a still point in the turning world.

Some breakthroughs are dramatic, but this one isn't because you are doing very little beyond welcoming yourself home. That's why Yoga is often described as the "journey of the return." You recognize that the world "in here" has all the qualities of home, which is very different from the stories we tell ourselves about hidden demons, dark forces, painful memories, and even the threat of going insane if we look too deeply inside. All these stories are banished when you follow the path laid out by Royal Yoga. Your inner world isn't a dark underground. Instead, it is the gateway to your true self. The so-called demons and dark forces are just another kind of *vritti* that blocks the light.

In Royal Yoga, you never fight or struggle against *vrittis*; you allow awareness to dissolve them, which happens by degrees. One of the most valuable secrets in Yoga is that it becomes easier, not harder, to dissolve the *vrittis* as you go deeper. *Pratyahara* teaches you to make the process of clearing out *vrittis* easier, beginning with the following exercise.

Exercise

The most basic practice in *pratyahara* is a full-body scan. Find a quiet place where you can lie down comfortably. Your bed or a soft rug will do. Lie on your back with your arms by your side. Closing your eyes, take a few deep breaths to relax.

Go inside and begin to scan your body, starting with your toes, feeling the experience as you move slowly and steadily toward your head. By *scan*, I mean letting your awareness sweep through you as you notice whatever comes to your attention. You might notice how hot or cold your body feels, how light or heavy, how pleasurable or uncomfortable a certain sensation might feel. Don't approach this exercise with any expectations. Using awareness to sweep your body is the sole thing you need to do.

Once you have finished your full-body scan, relax into the feeling of being comfortable inside yourself. This is the basic step that Yoga refers to as "withdrawal of the senses." You aren't focusing on what you might see, hear, touch, taste, or smell outside yourself. You are simply experiencing being "in here."

If you like, you can do a second scan, this time noticing the basic feeling of coming home. The qualities you are looking for were listed above as welcoming, familiar, safe, relaxing, happy, loving, and nurturing. To help yourself focus, it might help to recall a memory or image of a time when you felt welcomed, then let this feeling suffuse your body now. The same can be practiced with the other qualities. Use a memory of being safe, relaxed, happy, and so on. For some of these qualities, you probably won't need a memory. Just softly saying the word to yourself will bring up a matching feeling-sensation.

This exercise deepens the more often you practice it, and you will find it more and more enjoyable if you make it part of your daily routine.

TUESDAY

Seeds of Karma

Begin by silently repeating today's theme:

I set myself free from old memories.
I set myself free from old memories.

Royal Yoga shows you how to take control of your life, which strongly applies to karma. Most people are trapped in their past actions, which are the field of karma. This happens in a subtle, invisible way. Karma operates below the level of thoughts and feelings. To escape your karma, *pratyahara* shows you how to go to the level where karmic seeds are planted. The goal is to stop these seeds from sprouting. The principle is the same as weeding a garden. It is hard to pull up a full-grown weed, easier to pull up a weed that is just a seedling, and easiest of all to throw away the weed's seed before it has sprouted.

Karma is the Sanskrit word for "action," but it doesn't refer to every tiny thing you do or that your body does. Karmas are actions that leave a memory behind. Your first day at school, your first kiss, losing money at a casino, wrecking your car—these are memorable events. If a memory is strong enough, it can take charge of, color, or even control your life in various ways. A painful divorce colors your next relationship, for example. Because some events are painful to recall, memories of humiliation, defeat, failure, setbacks, and loss indicate the power that the past holds over us.

In the operation of karma, a positive memory can color or control your life, too. The high school quarterback who discovers that nothing in later life feels quite as good as being a teenage hero is overshadowed by a positive memory. Good or bad karma is how most people think of karma, but Royal Yoga is concerned with the binding power of all karmas, the stickiness that allows memories to color or control our lives.

In *pratyahara*, there are practical ways to achieve a state of awareness where you use your memories, instead of the other way around.

GAINING CONTROL OF YOUR MEMORIES

Don't believe everything you remember.

Substitute positive thoughts when a bad memory arises.

Don't dwell on the past.

Feel the fear but move ahead anyway.

If a memory throws you off, take time to center yourself.

Don't repeat the past just because your memory tells you to.

Practice being in the light through meditation.

Remind yourself that the only permanent reality is bliss.

The most untrustworthy memories arise from fear. Let's say you want to ask for a raise at work, but you remember that the last time you did that you were turned down. Memory is using you if this recollection is enough to stop you from asking for a raise; as a result, you defeat yourself. You can reverse the situation if you realize that today is new, which motivates you to go in and ask for a raise without being overshadowed by the past.

The practices for gaining control over your memories work as general guidelines for everyone, but they are most effective if you have a vision of constantly moving toward the light. Keep in mind that the light of pure awareness is the ultimate healer and that being in the light places you in the eternal now, which the past cannot touch.

Exercise

Pratyahara teaches that you can defuse your karma by starving it of attention. Attention is what makes karmic seeds sprout and grow. The earlier you detect them, the better. This ensures the least pain and struggle, and once you master the following exercise, there will be none at all.

Lie on your back, eyes closed, and take a few deep breaths. Place your attention in the region of your heart. Karma is easiest to detect as faint sensations and emotions in the heart. In an easy way, sense your heart becoming warm and relaxed. If it helps, you can visualize a warm, golden glow suffusing your heart.

As thoughts arise, they might draw your attention, which is only natural. As soon as you can, return to the warm glow of your heart. A thought or sensation might be unpleasant. Say to yourself, "I no longer need you," and resume the exercise. If a strong negative memory or feeling arises, open your eyes, take a few deep breaths, and let it subside. Then, once you feel more at ease in yourself, return to the exercise.

You can choose how long to perform this exercise. It works well for a few minutes or up to half an hour or more. But it would be best if you started with a shorter duration. If you are dealing with a painful memory, the attitude to take is that you can invite the memory to go. There is no reason for the past to linger over the present. All negative energy will dissipate once you learn how you are meant to use your memories, not the other way around.

WEDNESDAY

Exposing Three Myths

Begin by silently repeating today's theme:

I share one awareness with my body.
I share one awareness with my body.

By staying in the light, you begin to dissolve the separation of mind and body. The same creative intelligence flows through both. They share the same source in pure consciousness. The place that *pratyahara* leads you to is neither mind nor body, however. It is a silent field of awareness, and the faint sensations that arise in the field are like creative sparks or impulses.

It takes a shift in your perspective to fully inhabit this field of awareness. This is where you meet your true self. Any other version of yourself—physical, mental, social, or emotional—is secondary, a by-product of the flow of creative intelligence. There is no reason to judge yourself against these secondary selves. They spring from the one source that all of creation springs from. The problem is that we mistake them for who we really are. Then a set of false beliefs surrounds us and blocks the journey to the true self.

You will dispel your old conditioning and false beliefs by resting in the field of awareness; the light offers a feeling of bliss, oneness, and belonging that no secondary self can match. But Royal Yoga is also about knowledge (*vidya*) that contains truth, and truth, as the biblical adage says, can set you free.

To get closer to the truth about who you really are, let's examine its opposite. The opposite of truth is myth, and three powerful myths about mind and body pervade society.

Myth #1: You are captive inside your body.
Myth #2: You were created out of matter.
Myth #3: Your brain is doing the thinking.

These are such pervasive myths that you have probably never questioned them, but if we shatter each myth, you will come closer to merging your bodymind with the field of light. Only then will you experience who you really are.

Myth #1: You are captive inside your body.

Can you feel yourself inside your head looking out at the world, taking in its sights, sounds, tastes, smells, and textures? This is such a convincing experience that it is hard to fathom that it is false. But Royal Yoga teaches that it is. You aren't "in" your head or your body at all.

Your body is a zone of awareness, and your mind shares the same zone of awareness. *Pratyahara* teaches this fundamental truth.

When the two zones of awareness are separate, you can feel like a captive in your body because of pain, disease, and aging. The mind wants to escape from these experiences and is driven into separation as the only way out. But once you shatter the myth of being "in" your body, you realize that there is only one zone—the bodymind—sharing the same life. With this realization comes the ability to free yourself from being held hostage. Merged as one consciousness, you open the possibility that you are not your body or your mind. This realization frees you from pain and suffering and makes aging irrelevant. You grow into the truth that you are timeless, and, at the same time, bliss overwhelms any physical or mental pain.

Myth #2: You were created out of matter.

This myth was born out of the worldview that traces all of creation back to physical events, processes, and things. The thing can be as small as a quark, the event as titanic as the Big Bang. Worldviews are consistent, but that doesn't make them the truth. By showing you that you can experience yourself as one zone of awareness, *pratyahara* frees you from the trap of materialism. You begin to live the truth that consciousness is all-embracing.

Proving that this all-embracing consciousness exists (call it God or the gods, Buddha mind, Brahman) has vexed humanity for centuries, yet we can cut through all the confusion and conflict quite simply. The proof that consciousness underlies everything comes down to one thing: knowing. Nature knows what it is doing. If Nature were only random events that shuffled matter and energy around, it would know nothing, and existence would be meaningless. Yet every cell in your body knows how to sustain itself by organizing hundreds of thousands of chemical reactions per second. A cell isn't a bag of proteins suspended in a watery soup. It is organized intelligence. Every living thing is organized intelligence, and there is no reason to claim that this intelligence didn't precede life on Earth. The entire cosmos leading up to life on Earth is a sequence of events governed and controlled by creative intelligence.

Pratyahara teaches that you can also govern and control the events in your body because you are the same creative intelligence that lies at the heart of everything. The most advanced yogis achieve such an amazing degree of control that they can consciously lower vital functions like heart rate, breathing, and body temperature nearly to zero, as the yogi merges fully into the zone of awareness. The next step is to erase all physical limitations. Advanced yogis can experience being in two places simultaneously or even visiting other dimensions. Without exploring *pratyahara* that deeply, as Patanjali does in the *Yoga Sutras*, the issue of these advanced powers—*siddhis*—remains apart from everyday life. But you can achieve much more control over the physical than you realize, thanks to the freedom of awareness that humans are gifted with. At the very least, by accepting your body as a zone of awareness, you free it to heal, evolve, strengthen its immunity, and resist or reverse aging. Those processes occur in the one shared awareness of the bodymind.

Myth #3: Your brain is doing the thinking.

Turning the brain into a thinking organ is an offshoot of materialism. Whenever you are tempted to believe that your brain is the thinker, not you, look around. Is your TV making the actors in a movie do what they do? Has the piano in the corner learned how to play Bach? Does your computer know what you mean when you type a word? A television, a piano, and a computer are passive instruments waiting for consciousness to activate them. Likewise, it is pure illusion to claim that the brain can think.

The chemicals in a brain cell are the same as those in the skin cells of your big toe, and the functioning of brain cells differs very little from the functions of every other cell in the body. A three-pound lump of gray matter cannot escape its status as a batch of chemicals, and we mustn't attribute love, compassion, creativity, and so on to a batch of chemicals, either. The brain isn't even aware that it exists. Until the skull is opened to reveal it, there is no subjective experience that says, "Here I am. I am your brain."

Pratyahara teaches that your brain occupies the same zone of awareness as the rest of your body. Creative intelligence pours through every cell; a brain cell isn't exceptional. The creative intelligence in your immune system is assigned the tasks necessary to keep you healthy and protected from disease organisms. This intelligence is so complex that the immune system has been called a "floating brain," whose home is in the bloodstream and lymphatic system, which, by their very nature, are constantly in motion.

A brain cell stands out because its task is to transmit words, thoughts, impulses, desires, hopes, fears, and everything else associated with the mind. The brain itself has never had a thought. But when merged with the field of creative intelligence, the bodymind, the brain contributes to the wholeness of life. Oneness is all. If you claim that the mind creates the brain or that the brain creates the mind, neither statement is valid without the other being valid. This is a natural merging that gives Royal Yoga its basis in reality.

Exercise

The practices of *pratyahara* give you more control over your body, which begins by finding the control switch in your awareness. Lie comfortably on your back with your hand on your breastbone above the heart. Feel your heartbeat, then lift your hand away and sense your heartbeat in your body awareness alone.

You may have to repeat this a few times, but most people can easily sense a pulsation in the vicinity of the heart, and many can feel their actual heartbeat.

Now place your hands at your side and move the pulsing sensation to your fingertips. Feel the faint pulsation of the blood coursing through your fingers. This exercise shows you that you have more control over body awareness than you think. You can have the intention of your body feeling light or heavy, warm or cold, solid or hollow. With practice, you can intentionally make your heart rate and breathing slow down, and the intention will be enough to create these changes. But the whole process begins by showing yourself that you can merge into the zone of the bodymind and move your awareness wherever you want it to go.

THURSDAY

Magical Lies

Begin by silently repeating today's theme:

I vibrate in the field of light.
I vibrate in the field of light.

When *pratyahara* talks about withdrawing the senses, the main reason is to turn inward, but another reason is just as important: The senses cannot be trusted. Everyone has a glimmer of this since we all know, despite the evidence of our eyes, that the sun does not, in fact, rise in the morning and set at night. But Yoga goes much further, declaring that the five senses wrap us in a web of magical lies. You cannot be in touch with reality, including the reality of your true self, if you are under the spell of these lies.

Yoga describes the whole scheme of magical lies as *maya*, or "illusion," but I find that this terminology makes people uncomfortable. If this world is an illusion, then what are we supposed to cling to? The physical world and everything in it aren't going anywhere, no matter what Yoga says. Clearly, you can't live in the world and simultaneously call it a total lie—no one could psychologically endure such doublethink.

Pratyahara shows another way, which is based on an innocent-looking word that has amazing potency: *vibration*. Take any object—a tree, a dog, a skyscraper, or a molecule—and we can trace its origin to a set of vibrations. In quantum physics, these vibrations are described as "ripples in the quantum field." In Yoga, there are "ripples in consciousness." The fact that the cosmos is held together by invisible vibrations doesn't change everyday life, although it is an astonishing fact. But vibrations in consciousness *are* everyday life.

Pratyahara doesn't ask you to smash your way through the thickets of *maya*. Rather, you learn to choose the level of vibrations you want to identify with. Being the realm of the five senses, *maya* is a gross level of vibrations—at this level, rocks are hard, the wind is soft, roses smell sweet, garbage stinks. Thought is a subtler level of vibration, a realm of imagination, abstract concepts, and the whole scheme of wishes, dreams, fears, and memories that inhabit the mind.

Go one level deeper, and you are in the realm of *pratyahara*, where vibrations are born, emerging faintly from the unbounded field of your awareness the way that quarks emerge from the unbounded "quantum foam" that constantly hums and vibrates. Reality bubbles up like fizz in a carbonated drink. But this doesn't describe the way that every level of reality does a flip, completely overturning the level of reality next to it. At the level of *maya*, one experiences physical qualities, like hardness, solidity, warmth, and heaviness, and their opposites, which is why you can instantly distinguish a rock from a feather.

At the level of the mind, there is a flip, and physical qualities become imaginary. You can see a rock or a feather in your mind's eye, but they cannot be touched or weighed. This level is where most people stop, but there is another flip if you go deeper. Now the imaginary feather and the imaginary rock no longer exist, but the vibrations that give rise to them do. What is a feather without its light softness or a rock without its solid hardness?

Both dissolve into creative intelligence. The whole rationale behind *pratyahara* is that creative intelligence contains all the essentials for creating anything. To make this more personal, this is the level where you are created, with all your essential ingredients held in place, precisely as the essentials of a rock, feather, or any other object are held in place. In *pratyahara*, your essentials are very different from the body and mind you experience, yet you will still recognize yourself if you list these invisible ingredients.

THE "STUFF" THAT IS YOU

Your true essence is timeless, unborn, and undying.

Every atom of your body is an expression of creative intelligence.

Every choice you make reverberates throughout the field of pure consciousness.

You are embraced by the organizing power of the field, which governs and regulates everything.

You occupy a unique place in creation.

You are whole because the field is whole.

Human beings can see what they are made of and access their source in the timeless field of pure awareness. No one can explain this, the ultimate mystery known as self-awareness. Each of us is designed to be self-aware—it is simply a fact of human existence. The field of pure awareness is open to all. No one can be deprived of access to their source. At the same time, you can choose how self-aware you wish to be.

There is an almost complete absence of self-awareness at one extreme, which is marked by fear, denial, ignorance, unconscious behavior, and robotic conditioning. At the other extreme is *pratyahara*, immersing yourself in the light, which makes you self-aware in every moment. There is nothing more to seek or desire out of life. Placed in the flow of creative intelligence, you identify with your true self as naturally as you once identified with your five senses. You have broken the spell of *maya*. In place of magical lies, you experience your essence, and every gift of the light is yours for the taking.

Exercise

You were created from the unbounded field of pure awareness, which is your true source. To absorb what it means to be unbounded, sit quietly with eyes closed and take a few deep breaths. Once you feel centered and settled, direct your attention to the air as it passes in and out of your nose. Visualize each breath as a small puff of air. Now with the next out-breath, see the puff of air getting bigger, and with the next in-breath, see the air coming to you from a larger space.

Continue the process of expansion until you visualize inhaling air from the whole room and exhaling it into the whole room. If you are sitting by an open window, continue expanding, seeing air coming to you from the neighborhood, then the city, the countryside, never stopping until you visualize the planet giving you air with each in-breath and receiving the air back with each out-breath. (If your room doesn't have an open window or any windows at all, visualize an open window.)

A variation on this exercise is to visualize the expansion of light instead of air. Direct your attention to your heart. Visualize a dot of white light there. With each in-breath and out-breath, see the dot pulsate, gradually expanding, the same way you expanded the air going in and out of you.

Watch the pulsing light fill your body, then expand to fill the room, the neighborhood, and the city, until you can see pulsations of light coming to you in all directions without limit. These two exercises get you in touch with the infinite field that is your essence.

FRIDAY

Last Stop for Karma

Begin by silently repeating today's theme:

I allow the light to find me.
I allow the light to find me.

Every person has a double fate. We are destined to be embedded in *maya*—the scheme of magical lies driven by karma. That is our first fate. But we are also destined to live in the light. Both fates are necessary. Karma keeps the universe going, like a cosmic machine with an infinite number of moving parts, perfectly meshing together. Anything that requires moving parts, connections, and cause and effect comes under the purview of karma. The moving parts can be the chemicals rushing in and out of every cell; the connections can be the molecular bonds that keep these chemicals intact. At a subtler level, the moving parts can be your thoughts; the connections are the story you weave from these thoughts.

Out of habit, most people divide their karma along the lines of pleasure and pain; good karma makes life pleasant, while bad karma brings discomfort and suffering. But the real issue is karma itself. If you achieved a life of perfect pleasure without a hint of suffering, you would still be trapped inside the web of magical lies.

The second fate solves this dilemma. Karma no longer touches you when you live in the light. No other living creature (as far as we know) can consciously step out of the karmic machine. Unique on Earth, Homo sapiens can defy biological programming. If everyone knew this fact, Yoga would be the path chosen by all of humanity. There would be different motivations for this choice. The experience of bliss would entice some people; others would be drawn by the lure of freedom or the end of pain and suffering. These are obviously very desirable things, so why isn't Yoga central to everyone's life?

The most basic answer is that no one told us we had a second fate—the web of magical lies is the only reality we have ever experienced. A spider's web is gossamer; it snares its prey by being sticky. The web of magical lies has its own kind of stickiness. It is convincing. If you are convinced that the reality delivered by the five senses is real, you will be stuck for life. Yet, somehow, Yoga arose over the centuries as proof that getting stuck isn't inevitable.

The discovery that you can escape, win your freedom, and live in the light is personal—it is repeated one person at a time. Religion can sweep up masses of humankind in a vision of the divine, but Yoga isn't like that. You alone can go inside; you alone can experience the light; you alone can make higher consciousness your life's goal. When you do, karma has reached its last stop. The cosmic machinery, including the machinery of the body, will keep churning. Nothing can stop it, short of the death of the universe, and even that event might begin another cosmic cycle.

What karma is doing won't be your concern, however. You view it from a place that is timeless, unchanging, unborn, undying, and whole. This place can't be reached by karmic means. That is, you can't go anywhere, do anything, or think up a scheme to get there. If karma could bring you into the light, why hasn't it? Because that's not karma's purpose. You arrive at the light by realizing that it exists. Notice that the word *realize* has *real* inside it. To realize that you can be free of your karma, you must see the reality beyond the web of magical lies.

Pratyahara is the final turning inward that reveals everything. This is why it is considered a breakthrough. Your inner experiences all lead here, like all roads leading to Rome and all compasses showing true north. Each glimpse of the light points you in the right direction. We humans are designed to respond to love, compassion, truth, beauty, and the other qualities of the light. The karmic machinery is powerful, but it cannot stand up to the light; we instinctively prefer bliss to pleasure. The experience of love can overturn a whole life.

The great Bengali poet Rabindranath Tagore phrased it perfectly: "Love is the only reality, and it is not a mere sentiment. It is the ultimate truth that lies at the heart of creation." In the end, the light chooses you, instead of the other way around. Its appeal draws you closer and closer to your source. However, in *pratyahara*, there are vestiges of actions you can take that respond to the light.

HOW TO LET THE LIGHT CHOOSE YOU

Notice any glimpse of the light you experience.

Rest in the experience, letting it soak in.

Value these glimpses and feel grateful for them.

Sustain the light by devoting yourself to being conscious.

These steps aren't an agenda or a program. They are an attitude you take once you realize that you have a chance to escape your karma and the whole karmic machinery. To put it simply, having reached the threshold, it takes only the tiniest step to cross it.

Exercise

There is no effort involved to live in the light. If you have the right attitude, the light seeks you out and becomes the place you want to be. A little practice in adopting the right attitude is helpful, however. Sit quietly with your eyes closed, and let your mind go to a moment when you glimpsed the light. This could be a moment of love, truth, beauty, compassion, or blissfulness. Don't force your recollection. Once you have the intention, a memory will come to you. Sit easily, take a few deep breaths, and allow an image to arise.

Once it does, the memory will be very pleasant, but it will also tend to fade. While it is with you, rest in the feeling that surrounds it. Perhaps you envision seeing your child taking her first step or a beautiful sunset or an act of kindness that touched your heart. Remain with the feeling and quietly express your gratitude for it. Say to yourself, "Nothing is more real than this."

Let the warmth of the memory touch you the way the experience touched you. Sit quietly for a moment or two, breathing deeply before you get up and resume your day.

THE POWER OF ATTENTION

(Limbs of Yoga: *Dharana, Dhyana, Samadhi*)

THIS PART OF THE JOURNEY

Once you live in the light completely, the journey to find your true self comes to an end. But, from another perspective, life has just begun. The entire condition of separation is over, and new horizons open up.

In separation, you faced every day with either/or choices. The twin motivations of desire and fear were ever-present; if you made a wrong choice, things could easily spin out of control. At the very least, everyone's life was overshadowed by the unpredictable arrival of pain and suffering.

The last three limbs of Yoga are devoted to the ideal life that becomes possible once you have found your true self. I will treat all three limbs, known as *dharana, dhyana,* and *samadhi,* as one, because they are intimately joined. Taken together, they provide a map of life in wholeness. Each limb offers a necessary element if you want to find unity instead of separation.

Dharana enables you to pay attention so sharply that anything can be known.

Dhyana enables you to transcend all obstacles to experience higher consciousness.

Samadhi enables you to reach deeper and deeper levels of awareness.

At first glance, this trinity sounds abstract and otherworldly. In everyday life we don't think in such terms, being occupied with a constant stream of thoughts, feelings, sensations, and desires. You don't need to understand the workings of pure awareness. But the light is nothing but pure awareness and being able to navigate it opens the possibility of miracles, as we'll see in this final week.

MONDAY

The Source

Begin by silently repeating today's theme:

My life springs from pure awareness.
My life springs from pure awareness.

Everything must have a source and a starting point, whether it's the Big Bang that brought the universe into existence or the next thought you are about to have. Yoga brings us to the source of all things, including you and me.

But what is the source? That's not an easy question to answer. When you take a plane to another city, you get off the plane once you arrive at your destination. Royal Yoga also brings you to a new destination, but there is no airport or train station. No destination. What greets you at the source isn't anything describable, much less tangible.

Yet, somehow, for thousands of years, the source has been the most valuable attainment anyone can have. The last three limbs of Yoga allow you to verify this for yourself. *Dharana* puts you at the source and allows you to stay there effortlessly. *Dhyana* allows you to realize where you are. *Samadhi* enables you to sink deeper and deeper into the source, revealing its infinite scope. Does this description satisfy the mind of a seeker? Not really. Our minds crave words, sensations, and things we can grasp. But the source exists beyond the senses, beyond logic. To paraphrase the *Tao Te Ching*, the source that can be named is not the source.

Dharana shows you how to rest in the source while still leading a normal life. Both things are necessary to live at a state of higher consciousness. If you live a normal life without knowing your source, there is no escape from fear, doubt, and insecurity. At the same time, if you have contact with the source but no life, you will waste the infinite creative potential that flows from the source.

Dharana opens the way for exploring the source. Those who devote their lives to this are known as "seers." They spend their time witnessing the infinite play of consciousness, and, in that way, they reach fulfillment. How much time you devote to witnessing is up to you, but some features of the source are a given for everyone, as follows:

THE NATURE OF THE SOURCE

Pure, boundless existence.

Pure awareness, without the contents of thought.

Total absence of fear, including fear of death.

Infinite creative potential.

Pure bliss.

Truth with a capital "T."

Infinite dynamism.

An all-pervasive sense of unity.

Looking over this list, some people might assert that the source should be called God. At the very least, you might be suspicious that this is all pie in the sky. It is understandable that anyone might find talk about pure existence, infinite creative potential, and the rest of it utterly unbelievable. Without a fixed and fast connection with the source, you can't really tell.

The key words above are *fixed* and *fast*, because you are always connected to source. If you reread the list that describes the nature of the source, every item relates to your life here and now. You exist, you are dynamic. You feel inspired by creativity, you value the truth. The simplest way to explain the source is to call it the compressed concentration of the values we already live by. In separation, we experience fragments of love, compassion, truth, beauty, and creativity that turn out to be fleeting and temporary. But those fragments hint at an important truth, perhaps the most important: The source knows us and wants us to know it.

Exercise

You can get a feeling for being at the source with a simple exercise. Sit quietly with your eyes closed. Once you feel relaxed, try not to exist. Interpret this challenge any way you wish. You can imagine not existing before you were born or never existing again after you die. You can visualize yourself being vaporized or dissolving into nothingness. This is not an exercise in the macabre. It does, however, demonstrate that no matter what tactic you choose or how intently you pursue your imagined non-existence, you can't stop existing. "To be or not to be" isn't an option.

No matter how terrible or glorious life seems to be, two elements accompany you hand in hand. There is existence, and there is the flow of creative intelligence that provides experiences. Once these elements are compressed and concentrated to the utmost, you will be at the source.

TUESDAY

Going Beyond

Begin by silently repeating today's theme:

My essence is transcendent.
My essence is transcendent.

The last three limbs of Yoga are like a tripod, held up by three legs. The first leg, *dharana*, gives you a fulfilling life while you simultaneously remain at the source. The second leg is *dhyana*, usually described as "meditation." That's not very helpful, however, since *meditation* is a vague, amorphous term that we apply in all kinds of situations. Basically, when someone dwells inwardly on any idea, feeling, or experience, they can call that a meditation. But in Royal Yoga, *dhyana* is "transcendence," going beyond the limits of everyday experience.

In its most basic form, transcendence is a very common experience. If you are a mother with a cranky baby who won't stop crying, you don't cry, too (unless, maybe, you are completely exhausted). You transcend the baby's crankiness to find out what the real issue is—the child might need sleep, food, or a change of diaper. Without the ability to transcend daily experience, humans would never have evolved. We can stand aside from our own actions, analyze them, and move forward to new and unexplored territory. By the route of inquiry and discovery, the human mind transcends itself.

Yet the mind can't take full credit for transcending. Your mind is constantly wrapped up in thoughts and feelings. If Yoga hadn't pointed out the possibility of *dhyana*—transcending to a much deeper level—people would be confined to the mind's endless activity, as, indeed, countless people are. The original seers of Yoga, who are nameless and lost to ancient history, realized that there is one element common to all thoughts, which is awareness. This commonality can be seen when we notice that a gold watch, a gold spoon, and a gold coin look totally different, but all are made of gold. Gold is each item's essence. Your essence is awareness.

There are signposts to know if you are indeed cultivating a relationship with awareness. You know that you are on the right path when:

> You go inside for answers.
> You reflect on your thoughts.
> You contemplate a new possibility.
> You have an insight.
> You experience an "aha" moment.
> You look for inner peace and quiet.
> You get a glimpse of wonder.
> You feel a sudden impulse of joy.
> You are filled with love.

These experiences are momentary, fleeting hints that transcendence is yours to master. On the flip side, there are signs that tell us we are moving around in circles, which leads to dizziness and confusion. Unfortunately, these unaware states are also common, and you experience them when:

You feel stressed.

You are distracted and scattered.

You feel depressed.

You get lost in worry and anxiety.

You crave escapism.

You are tense and can't relax.

What these two lists tell us is that we spend our lives bouncing between two states, between awareness and its opposite. If you swing too far from awareness, your life will be dominated by routine and habit, the same old same old. Yet even if you are fortunate enough that this hasn't happened to you, it is a genuine discovery to realize that you experience transcendence in everyday life. The meditative state isn't reserved for a special time of day, set apart for closing your eyes and performing a meditation practice. Life can be spent in a form of total meditation.

No meditation practices would ever work if *dhyana* weren't a natural tendency of the human mind. To love, create, be kind, act selflessly, experience wonder, and feel inspired are totally human and natural. They are made possible by *dhyana*, the impulse to transcend. Once this sinks in, Royal Yoga is here to teach that going beyond is boundless. You can transcend so completely that you reach your source and merge with your true self.

Exercise

Behind every experience there is awareness, which you can locate anytime you wish. To show yourself how this works, try the following: Sit back and look around you. Focus on any object—a table lamp, a chair, a paperweight, the sky outside. Now tune it out by allowing your eyes to go into soft focus while you move your attention to the center of your chest. Now go back and forth. See the object, then go inward and tune it out. Repeat for a minute or two.

The process is simple, and you might have your own way of moving your attention inward. Regardless of how you do it, what we call "tuning out" moves your attention and shifts your focus, which is the critical element in meditation. Once you feel familiar with how to turn your attention inward, you know how to transcend. This is useful whenever you find yourself in an unaware state, such as feeling stressed, distracted, worried, or scattered. Look at an object, put your eyes in soft focus, and move your attention to your heart. By going beyond, you strengthen the habit of being aware until it becomes just as natural as being unaware.

WEDNESDAY

Being Here

Begin by silently repeating today's theme:

I am grounded in life's infinite potential.
I am grounded in life's infinite potential.

The eighth limb of Yoga, known as *samadhi*, is about being present, right here, right now, with as much awareness as possible. You can think of *samadhi* as a deep dive into a state of silent awareness. It is an experience of stillness amid the chaos around you.

But you and I crave experiences. We crave a little of the chaos, as does everyone. So what does *samadhi* mean to us? Imagine Albert Einstein stretched out on a sofa taking a nap. He isn't thinking about physics; he looks like anyone else taking a nap. But even asleep he has the awareness of a genius, and the potential for great thoughts will be activated once more when he wakes up. In other words, take away any single thought, and what remains is far more valuable: the potential for deep awareness.

When you hear a voice in your head, its loudness or softness doesn't indicate how deep or expanded your awareness is. If you are new to playing a musical instrument and you think, "I will play the piano," the result is going to be very different than if a famous virtuoso thinks, "I will play the piano." The difference is determined by *samadhi*, meaning that it takes practice to reach this level. Some fish stay near the surface of the ocean; others live in its darkest depths. Likewise, your thoughts float up from the level of awareness you have attained and often this is the result of how much you practice going in and out of these transcendent states.

The benefits of *samadhi* are revealed only through personal experience. As your *samadhi* deepens through meditation, the following changes appear:

THE GIFTS OF *SAMADHI*
You are able to detect an underlying bliss in everything.
You appreciate your life more fully.
You gain satisfaction simply by being here.
You settle into silent awareness easily.
The outer world no longer dominates your life.

Mood swings decrease dramatically, bringing fewer highs and lows. You feel secure in who you are.

Though Royal Yoga bestows upon us priceless gifts, they are not entirely welcome by the ego-personality, which thrives on emotional drama, a constant stream of desires, a restless search for distraction, and an avoidance of pain and fear. You can easily be persuaded that this whole setup is preferable to the boring sameness of silent awareness. But that's a false conclusion. The deeper your *samadhi*, the more fulfilling your existence becomes. You don't have to change any aspect of your outer life. Every experience, large or small, allows the light of awareness to shine through.

Exercise

No matter what you happen to be doing or thinking, you are floating at some level of *samadhi*. This isn't something people are normally aware of, but you can experience your level of awareness with the following exercise. Make a list of three things you like, three things you like a lot, and three things you deeply love. Perhaps a TV sitcom or a peanut butter cookie is something you like, while going to the beach or playing chess is something you like a lot, and your child or the music of Bach is something you deeply love.

Whatever you wrote down, you went to a different level of awareness to make your choices. You can verify this by taking each item of your list, shutting your eyes, and experiencing it inside as an image or feeling. The intensity of something you casually like will be shallow compared to the intensity of something you deeply love.

Therefore, simply by being here, which is common to everyone, you are expressing the infinite possibilities of human awareness. This is what *samadhi* is here to show you.

THURSDAY

Three-in-One

Begin by silently repeating today's theme:

I am the creator of my personal reality.
I am the creator of my personal reality.

Each limb of Yoga gives you more control over some aspect of your life, beginning with social interactions, emotions, ingrained conditioning, thoughts, and, finally, your level of awareness. But just as a book on anatomy is nothing like a living body, we don't dissect our lives and place each aspect in its own pigeonhole. Royal Yoga teaches you how to practice control over this and that, but the whole enterprise would be useless unless it came together in complete mastery, the way a music student practices exercises until the day arrives when she is a full-fledged artist, a master of her instrument.

The last three limbs of Yoga draw everything together, bringing you to full mastery. The term for full mastery is *samyama*, which means to "bind" or "tie together" in Sanskrit. *Samyama* is necessary because it unites the last three limbs of Yoga into one process. The process can be dissected into three parts as we have seen—*dharana, dhyana,* and *samadhi*—but they are bound together and inseparable, which is why they are referred to as a three-in-one. (Unwittingly, the Three Musketeers hit upon this in their cry of "One for all, and all for one.")

Further, common experience tells us that there have to be three elements in every experience: a knower, the object known, and the process of knowing. Right now, you, the knower, are reading these words, which are the object of knowledge, while the act of reading is the process of knowing. You can remove the word *reading* and substitute *seeing and hearing*. The five senses contain the same three elements. To smell the fragrance of a rose requires a perceiver to bend over it, the fragrance that wafts to his nose, and the process of inhaling and absorbing the delicious fragrance.

Why do these three elements mean so much if they are present all the time? Here lies the deepest secret of Royal Yoga. If knower, known, and process of knowing are separate, your whole life will be led in separation, but if they are united as three-in-one, then you have attained unity. You have reached the womb of creation, and from here you can create your own reality any way you choose. That's a breathtaking possibility, which is the main reason it takes the eight limbs of Yoga to get there. Becoming the creator of your personal reality is too far a reach unless you approach it one step at a time.

On our journey we've encountered the countless drawbacks and problems that arise from living in separation. Let me offer a brief reminder of them.

In separation, the *vrittis*, or mental obstacles, block the light.
Outer events overshadow your life.
Moods and emotions pull you this way and that.
The constant restless activity of the mind is inescapable.
Maya throws up a screen of illusion.
The stream of either/or choices never ends.
Karma, the residue of the past, limits what you can do in the present.

In an ideal life, none of these drawbacks and limitations exist. They vanish because what created them in the first place—the state of separation—

has vanished. In Royal Yoga there is one healing for all. It consists in reaching unity consciousness, which is another way of expressing the state of three-in-one. I must underscore that unity consciousness isn't exotic, mystical, or out of reach. Every time you have an experience, the three elements of knower, known, and process of knowing automatically come together. The difference with *samyama* is that you are aware of what's going on and can control it.

To put it another way, existence can take care of itself. If you think, feel, and act from a deeper, more expanded level of awareness, everything you would like to control is able to take care of itself. You are the co-creator of your reality, however, not its sole creator. That role belongs to creative intelligence as it flows in, around, and through you.

Exercise

As you undertake the practices of Royal Yoga, you correct the difficulties that arise from living in separation until they are gone entirely. Unity consciousness is built from small steps; it dawns as a completely unique state all its own. Glimpses of it are given in rare experiences we call "epiphanies" and "revelations," which come of their own accord and are totally unpredictable. We have no control over them, and no exercise can duplicate one.

However, you can promote your evolution to unity consciousness by taking time to read about someone else's epiphany. The New Testament, the Sufi poetry of Rumi, and the ecstatic poems of Rabindranath Tagore were my first touchstones of epiphany, and I still turn to them regularly. They provide inspiration of a special kind by conveying a taste of what unity consciousness feels like. Vicarious revelation has its own genuine feeling of transcending the everyday world and going into the light.

Today take a little time to inspire yourself by going back to your own touchstones, the things that have helped you to realize that there is more to life than just material experience. Whether the source is scripture, poetry, music, or a movie, the test is for you to allow yourself to enter into, say, a Mozart concerto or a ballad by Alicia Keys, and experience transcendence. Let go and be present in the notes, in the rhythms, in the harmonies. Allow someone else's epiphany to reach out and touch you. Such experiences provide a foretaste of what unity consciousness is like all the time.

FRIDAY

The First and Last Mystery

Begin by silently repeating today's theme:

I embody the field of infinite possibilities.
I embody the field of infinite possibilities.

Royal Yoga begins and ends with the same mystery. One can call it the mystery of existence, but, to make it more personal, this is the mystery of "Who am I?" Choosing your identity is up to you. Every action you take is rooted in who you think you are. If you spend money freely, this reflects a belief that you are rich (which might or might not be true). String together the tags and labels that apply to you, and they give a shorthand account of your identity. "I am Deepak, a doctor born in India, married with a wife and two children" is a string of labels and tags that apply to me, and I can add many more, as many as I wish.

People spend their entire lives desiring "good" labels like rich, powerful, loved, attractive, and young, while hoping that "bad" labels don't stick to them, including poor, weak, stupid, dishonest, and unlovable. This is how life works in separation. But tags and labels can't possibly describe what it means to be fully human, and only a fully human answer to "Who am I?" will be truly satisfying.

Royal Yoga teaches that you are the true self—we've established that much so far—but what are the actions of the true self? What can it do that those other selves cannot?

WHAT YOUR TRUE SELF CAN DO
It can fulfill all desires.
It can banish all pain and suffering.
It can give the experience of eternity.
It can show you the reality of boundless Being.
It can be anywhere and everywhere at once.
It can open the way to every state of higher consciousness.

These are absolute statements. There is a quantum leap from fulfilling one desire and fulfilling all desires, and the same applies when healing one cause of pain and suffering and healing all pain and suffering. Because it is absolute, the true self isn't anything like the other selves you can identify with. In separation, you experience limits and boundaries; you have no trouble knowing what is "me" and what is "not me." But all opposites vanish in unity consciousness. Looking around, you see the light extending infinitely in all directions, and *you are the light*.

This isn't a mystical statement. In physics there is a point, known as a "singularity," from which the universe springs. The singularity is so small it cannot be measured, like the period at the end of a sentence reduced to the vanishing point yet somehow still here. Time and space emerge from the singularity; therefore, it is neither here nor there. You can't locate it now, before, or after. Trillions of galaxies are contained in it, yet there is no "in" or "out" when it comes to the singularity itself.

The singularity is literally mind-boggling. The human mind can't conceive of the universe being contained in an infinitesimal point (although poets can imagine this, as in William Blake's famous lines: "To see a World in a Grain of Sand / And a Heaven in a Wild Flower / Hold Infinity in the palm of your hand / And Eternity in an hour").

Yoga has its own word for a singularity: *bindu*, which just means "point." The *bindu* is a point of awareness that contains every possible experience available to a human being. Like a singularity, the *bindu* can't be measured—it is too small to have a dimension in time and space—and yet it contains an infinity of possibilities. The best, simplest, and truest way to know who you are is here. You are a point of awareness from which all possibilities flow outward.

With this realization comes the big payoff. The *bindu*, a mere point of awareness, is where *samyama* operates. *Samyama*, as we saw, unites knower, known, and process of knowing. If you can control *samyama*, you can have any experience you want. All the stories about supernatural powers attained by yogis, swamis, and saints are extensions of *samyama*. To Patanjali, walking on a sunbeam is as natural as walking through a meadow. This isn't something you are asked to believe or not to believe. It is something you are asked to explore.

Now you know who you are and the purpose of your life, as revealed by Royal Yoga. You are the creative source of your own reality, and your purpose is to explore how far your creative powers can take you. Once you get to the heart of the matter, life has only two phases. The first phase is spent in separation, the second phase in unity consciousness. One phase is fragmentary, the other is whole. The secret of existence, as revealed by Yoga, is that wholeness is in charge, even when you feel alone, weak, insignificant, and helpless. Awareness is in charge. Royal Yoga helps you to live this truth.

Explore this: Your true self is as indestructible as existence itself. Your creative power is untouched by any event in the outside world. As you wander through life, the truth about who you are seems to change as the scenery changes. Birth, death, and everything in between are controlled by *maya*, yet *maya* is contained by the *bindu*, a single point from which all of creation flows. Illusion may be part of experience, but awareness helps us to see illusion for what it really is, a parlor trick of the ego.

Exercise

Even though unity consciousness may feel as if it were far away, you can identify your true essence right now. Sit quietly, and when you feel settled, look around you. Notice what is in front of you, what is to the right, and what is to the left.

Now close your eyes and see the color blue in your mind. Open your eyes and look forward. Close your eyes, see the color blue again, then open your eyes and look to your right. Repeat and look to your left. Did the color blue move right, left, or center? No, even as the scenery changed, the color blue kept still and was motionless. It springs from the *bindu*, the still point that is your essence.

You can repeat this exercise with any quality you choose. Hum a tune to yourself. Look right and left. Did the tune move? Look outside the window as far as you can see, even up to the stars. Did the still point travel outside you? The *bindu* is always here and now. It has no properties. You can't assign any quality to it, like hot or cold, high or low, young or old. The *bindu* is your portion of eternity; it is where you stand in infinity. This is the first and last mystery of existence. The entire teaching of Royal Yoga comes down to "the still point of the turning world," as the poet T. S. Eliot put it. Now you are ready to launch yourself into the discovery of infinite possibilities that has always been your birthright.

PART II

By Sarah Platt-Finger

THE ASANAS

———

WHAT IS YOGA?

As Deepak alluded to earlier, the word *yoga* comes from the root word *yuj*, meaning to "harness," "yoke," or "unite." Simply put, yoga merges the disparate parts of the self into one unified state of awareness, allowing us to live fully in the light. There are many paths to that state of wholeness, and asana is one limb of the tree that makes up the yogic path. Yoga dates back more than five thousand years to India. The ancient teachings of yoga originate from the Vedas, an ancient Hindu scripture that disseminates the insights of the *rishis*, or seers, of India. These spiritually awakened aspirants interpreted the wisdom of the universe through Nature and its elements. According to the *rishis*, the human body is a vehicle that enables us to access a greater field of intelligence. The individual spirit is the microcosm of that intelligence, just like a drop of water is to the ocean. When a drop of water merges back into the ocean, it loses its form, shape, and identity. It becomes the ocean. The same is true for individual consciousness: When the soul, or *jiva atman*, merges with the ocean of intelligence, or Brahman, yoga happens.

The *Bhagavad Gita*, the great Indian epic from the *Mahābhārata*, translates *yoga* as "skill in action." The organization of our body as conscious action is asana.

WHAT IS ASANA?

The word *asana*, meaning "seat of awareness," is formally introduced in *The Yoga Sutras of Patanjali*, which was written and compiled sometime around 400–500 CE. The word *asana* is only referenced three times in the *Yoga Sutras*: once as part of the eight limbs of *ashtanga yoga* (sutra 2.29) and twice as a reference to *sthiram sukham* asana: asana as a steady, comfortable seat (sutra 2.46, 2.47). About a millennium later, Svātmārāma compiled the *Hatha Yoga Pradipika*. In this classic text, eighty-four asanas, most of which are seated, are referenced as postures for purification, optimal health, and vitality.

In the West, we have adapted asana to reflect the entire spectrum of yoga, when, really, it is only one aspect of it. The other seven limbs—*yama, niyama, pranayama, pratyahara, dharana, dhyana,* and *samadhi*—are also integral pathways to the experience of yoga. In this section, we are putting a lens on the limb of asana as a gateway to the light of pure consciousness.

The body is so much more than a shape; it is a process. Asanas are shapes that we make with our physical body to tap into this process, to tap into this state of awareness. But why do different shapes impact us differently? For some of us, one shape might feel glorious, while for others it might feel like torture. The answer lies in the unseen realm.

THE *SHARIRAS*

According to the ancient teachings of yoga, human existence is experienced through three bodies of energy, known as the *shariras*.

- The *sthula sharira* is the physical body, which consists of the body's muscles, bones, joints, and fluids. It is the densest energy body and is experienced through the senses.
- The *sukshma sharira* is the subtle body, which includes the 72,000 channels of energy that map our body, known as the *nadis*, as well as the chakra system, nerves, prana, thoughts, and feelings. The *sukshma sharira* can be felt but not measured.
- The *karana sharira* is the causal body. This consists of our karma, or the force that brought us into manifestation, and our spirit, the *jiva atman*. The *karana sharira* exists in pure potentiality and can only be accessed when we transcend the mind.

It is important to remember that, although we separate the *shariras* into three different bodies, they are integrally connected with each other. We can access the causal body from the physical, and we can also access the physical from the causal. When we practice yoga asanas, we move through these different densities of energy and can tap into the subtle energetic forces that govern us.

THE CHAKRAS

The word *chakra* in Sanskrit means "wheel" or "circle." Just as the Earth's rotation creates electromagnetic fields of energy, so, too, do these vortices of energy that run along the spine within our bodies. The chakras lie in our subtle body, but they govern our physical body and are governed by our causal body. There are seven main chakras, and the first five are essentially the headquarters of the elements that exist within us, known as the *maha bhutas*. They are earth, water, fire, air, and space.

In addition to its elemental quality, each chakra has a sound, shape, color, energy, and physical location in the body. They also have a front and a back gate, represented by the front and the back of the body, which we will explore later in this book. For our present purposes, we are most interested in the physical location and the energetic qualities associated with each chakra:

Chakra	Element	Location	Body Parts Associated with Chakra	Energetic Qualities
Muladhara (Root center)	Earth	Base of the spine	Feet, legs, pelvic floor, bowel	Grounded, steady, connected to survival needs, healthy boundaries
Svadishthana (Abode of self)	Water	In front of the sacrum, below the navel	Pelvis, bladder, reproductive organs	Creative, spontaneous, flexible, connected to sensuality and sexuality
Manipura (City of gems)	Fire	Navel center	Lumbar spine, abdomen, digestive organs	Empowered, brave, process-oriented, autonomous, healthy sense of self
Anahata (Unstruck)	Air	Center of the chest	Thoracic spine, rib cage, diaphragm, heart, lungs, shoulder girdle, arms, hands	Balance, harmony, connection, empathy, intimacy, unconditional love

Chakra	Element	Location	Body Parts Associated with Chakra	Energetic Qualities
Vishuddha (Purification center)	Space	Throat	Cervical spine, shoulder girdle, arms, hands, throat, jaw, tongue, ears	Clear communication with the universe and others, ability to be in silence, resonance
Ajna (Command center)	Light	In between eyebrows and slightly above	Eyes, forehead, brain	Imagination, clear vision, innovation, intuition, insight
Sahasrara (Crown chakra)	None	Top fontanel	Top fontanel, back crown (*bindu*)	Faith, trust, surrender, transcendence, liberation, embodiment

THE *GUNAS*

The *gunas* are the qualities of Nature that exist in all of matter. The quality of a rock, which is heavy, solid, and unmoving, is very different from the quality of a river, which is active, flowing, and constantly changing. We can see these different qualities play out in the natural world around us and experience them within us. The three *gunas* are: *rajas*, volition or desire; *tamas*, inertia; and *satva*, homeostasis.

The *gunas* manifest in the subtle body via the chakras. Each chakra can have either a positive charge, which activates and enlivens its qualities (*rajas*), or a negative charge, which soothes and reduces those qualities (*tamas*). When we are in balance in a particular chakra, it is in a state of harmony, or *satva guna*.

We also experience the *gunas* in the physical body, via the breath and our posture.

Let's look at the *gunas* and how they manifest in the physical body:

- *Rajas* manifests in the front of the body. It involves inhalation and is the force that literally projects our bodies forward into the future. When we stretch the front of the body, we open the chakras' front gate, which positively charges them and enhances their energetic qualities. By opening the front of the body, we externalize our energy. This stimulates a sense of extroversion and promotes connection to others.

- *Tamas* manifests in the back of the body. It is ushered in by the exhalation and is the force that connects us to the past. When we stretch the back of the body, we open the back gate of the chakras, which negatively charges the *gunas* and reduces their energetic qualities. By opening the back of the body, we internalize our energy and create a space for introspection and introversion, enhancing a sense of intimacy with ourselves.

- *Satva* manifests along the central line of the spine, known as *brahma nadi*. *Brahma nadi* is the energetic streak of intelligence that connects our lower consciousness to our higher consciousness. It can guide us to either manifestation or liberation, depending on the direction in which we move our energy along it. *Satva guna* is revealed when we balance the breath in and the breath out. It is present in the pauses between our thoughts and our connection to the present moment. When we balance the front and back of the body, and come into our own personal alignment, we bring the qualities of the chakras into harmony as well. This enables us to rest in our awareness without attachment, judgment, or projection into the future.

THE BREATH

Our breath is our source of life. It sustains us and all the functions in our body without us even trying. It is also the bridge that connects the mind and the body. If we want to know how we are feeling in the present moment, we must listen to our breath. When we breathe in longer than we breathe out, it usually indicates nervousness or anxiety. When we breathe out longer than we breathe in, it means we are feeling unmotivated or lethargic. When our breath is loud and effortful, it means that we are in a state of anger or tension. When our breath is quiet, it means that we are relaxed and at peace. Our breath directly reflects how we feel, but we can also change how we feel by changing our breath.

The breath is also the carrier of prana, the life force energy that enlivens and animates us. Prana is the electricity that rides on oxygen. It feeds all the functions in our body and works directly with the mind. Prana is an electrical current that travels through the subtle energy channels in the body, known as the *nadis*. We say that where your awareness goes is where the prana flows. When the prana flows freely through the *nadis*, we experience *sukha*, or ease. When there is an obstruction to the flow of prana, we experience *dukha,* or suffering.

What is a full, complete breath?

Many of us have imbalances in our breath because we do not know how to breathe. As Deepak mentioned earlier, the yogis measure life not by the number of years we live but by the number of breaths we take. By extending our breath, they believe, we are also extending our life span and the quality of our life.

Anatomically, this is what happens on a full, complete breath:

- On inhalation, the brain triggers the diaphragm muscles to contract. This flattens the diaphragm as the intercostal muscles between the ribs lift the rib cage out and up. The muscles along the spine contract to lift the sternum. The upper abdominal muscles relax, allowing the abdominal organs to press down into the abdominal cavity. All of this creates a vacuum in the chest, which makes air suck into the lungs. For a full, complete breath, the third, fourth, and fifth ribs are lifted by the pectoral muscles, and the scalene muscles lift the first two ribs on either side of the neck. These accessory breathing muscles are there for us to take in more air when we need it.

- On the exhalation, the reverse of this process happens. The neck, pectoral, intercostal, spinal, and diaphragm muscles all relax. This allows the flow of air out of the chest cavity. The lower abdominal muscles pull back in toward the body's center for the final expulsion of air.

When practicing asanas, we want to ensure that the architecture of the pose facilitates the anatomy of the breath. Some poses will compress the diaphragm, rib cage, belly, or chest. In each posture, we want to adjust our body to accommodate a full complete breath. This ensures the circulation of prana throughout the body.

Ujjayi Breath

It is optimal to breathe in and out through the nostrils to keep the breath long, slow, and controlled when practicing asanas. *Ujjayi*, or "victorious" breath, is a technique that involves narrowing the vocal cords at the back of the throat. This process slows down the passage of air in the pharynx, which lengthens and extends the breath. It also creates a warming effect on the breath, which helps build mental heat and focus. *Ujjayi* makes a whispery-like sound that stimulates the vagus nerve (the longest and most complex cranial nerve, a central part of the parasympathetic nervous system). *Ujjayi* gives our mind something audible to anchor to in each pose.

How to practice *ujjayi* breath:

- Inhale through your nostrils.
- As you exhale, open your mouth, and breathe out as if you were fogging up a mirror. Listen to the ocean-like sound of the breath and go to the very bottom of the exhalation.
- Now inhale and engage those same muscles at the back of the throat as you did on the exhalation, keeping your mouth open.
- Exhale again as if you were fogging up a mirror. Close your mouth halfway and breathe out through the nostrils, listening for that whispery-like sound of the breath. It should be audible just to you.
- Keep your mouth closed as you inhale through the nostrils.
- Continue to breathe slowly in and out like this, engaging the *ujjayi* breath.

The *Vayus*

The *vayus* are winds or directions of energy that govern the healthy functioning of our body. Each asana has a particular *vayu* or *vayus* that are dominant when we experience it. Each *vayu* has an element associated with it, a pattern of movement, and a specific function that it carries out. For example, when we practice an asana that activates the core, we elicit the qualities of digestion or conversion, which is *samana vayu*. When we open the chest, we encourage oxygen absorption into the body, which is *prana vayu*. The five *vayus* and their qualities are:

Vayu	Element	Function	Area of the Body
Apana	Earth	Elimination; downward flow	Feet, legs, pelvis
Vyana	Water	Circulation, distribution	All over
Samana	Fire	Conversion, metabolism	Navel
Prana	Air	Absorption, inspiration	Chest and head
Udana	Space	Projection, upward flow	Throat

The *Bandhas*

The Sanskrit word *bandha* means to "lock." When we perform *bandhas*, we are rechanneling our energy, the way a dam may redirect the flow of a river. We usually practice the *bandhas* on breath retentions, especially during *pranayama*. However, *bandhas* can be used in the asanas as well. They help us to create a dynamic state of grace that can empower us in our everyday life.

Here are the four *bandhas* and their functions:

- *Mula bandha* is the "root lock," located at the pelvic floor between the tailbone and the pubic bone. When we engage *mula bandha*, we lift the muscles of the pelvic floor, like an elevator, toward the navel. *Mula bandha* inhibits the downward flow of *apana* so that the upward energy—*udana*—can be integrated into the body. This helps us to feel our own presence and power in the postures.

- *Uddiyana bandha* means to "fly upward." It is the act of drawing the lower abdominal muscles back and up toward the spine, usually at the bottom of the exhalation. *Uddiyana bandha* stimulates *samana vayu*, and encourages energy to flow upward to the crown, especially during breath and meditation practices. Engaging a slight *uddiyana bandha* in the asana helps us engage our core, enabling us to contain our energy, rather than dispersing it.

- *Jalandhara bandha* means "net lock," and it is located at the neck and throat. When we perform *jalandhara bandha*, we draw the chin gently down toward the chest. This can be done on the retention of the inhalation or the exhalation during *pranayama* and meditation practices. *Jalandhara bandha* allows the upward energy, *udana*, to be directed back down along the central channel of the spine. *Jalandhara* stimulates the parasympathetic nerves at the brain stem, which cultivates a sense of calm and tranquility when practiced with the asanas.

- *Treta bandha* means "triple lock," and it involves the engagement of all three *bandhas* simultaneously. When the downward energy of *apana* moves up in *mula bandha*, and the upward energy of *udana* moves down in *jalandhara bandha*, they create friction, or *samana*, at the center of the spine, which helps to break our mental patterning and false identities. *Treta bandha* is useful when practicing arm balances, four-limbed poses, and inversions, as we seek to become more compact and buoyant. *Treta bandha* helps us to defy both gravity and the limited beliefs that weigh us down.

MUDRA

A *mudra* is a seal or a gesture that creates a circuit of energy in the body. *Mudras* are typically performed with the hands; however, they can also be done with the head, perineum, and through different shapes we create with the entire body. These gestures are powerful tools to shift our consciousness. Two *mudras* that we will explore in the asanas are *ashvini mudra* and *vajroli mudra*, both of which are performed in the perineum.

- *Ashvini mudra* involves engaging the anal sphincter muscles, which we use when we are inhibiting flatulence. When we perform *ashvini mudra* during forward bends, it creates a natural lift in the front of the body, which lengthens the spine and takes us out of *tamas* into *satva guna*.
- *Vajroli mudra* works the urethral sphincter muscles, which are the muscles we use to restrain the act of urination. When we perform *vajroli mudra* during backbends, it lifts the back of the body and takes us out of *rajas* into *satva guna*.

KRIYA

A *kriya* is an act to purify our consciousness. Many types of *kriya* are used in various methodologies for varying purposes. Through breath, sound (mantra), and visualization, we can light up our consciousness in a way that alters our experience in our body and in the pose itself. These two *kriyas* are particularly effective at enhancing our vitality in the asanas:

So Hum Kriya

Through our breath, we use this *kriya* to integrate the unbounded, universal intelligence into the physical body, making it manifest. This *kriya* allows us to receive pure potential with every breath in and embody that pure potential with every breath out. It is replenishing, rejuvenating, and inspiring.

How-to

Visualize a line of energy from the base of the spine to the crown of the head. This is *brahma nadi*, the cosmic superhighway that connects us to infinite intelligence.

As you breathe in, feel the ribs, the lungs, and the side of the body expand. Sense an electromagnetic field of energy entering through the crown of the head. Then observe the energy traveling down the central channel of the spine, to the space just in front of the sacrum, known as *kunda*.

As you breathe out, feel the lower belly retract. Imagine distributing that magnetism from in front of your sacrum out into each cell of your body, and feel your joints becoming spacious.

As you breathe in, silently hear the sound *so*, which is the sound of pure consciousness.

When you breathe out, silently hear the sound *hum*, the sound of transformation.

Integrate this *so hum* technique with each breath, reorienting your awareness to the subtle line of energy in each pose.

AROHAN AWAROHAN KRIYA

Arohan awarohan translates to "ascending descending," corresponding to the two main passages in the body: the front, which is *rajas*, and the back, which is *tamas*. It is also known as the "figure-8 breath" because of the route it follows in the body. When we practice *arohan awarohan*, not only are we are balancing the front and the back gates of the physical body and, therefore, the chakras, we are also bringing coherence to the breath and our energy fields. It is a powerful action that brings us back to *satva guna*—the state of pure being.

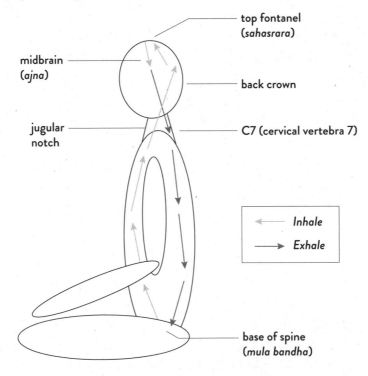

top fontanel
(*sahasrara*)

midbrain
(*ajna*)

back crown

jugular
notch

C7 (cervical vertebra 7)

⟵ *Inhale*

⟶ *Exhale*

base of spine
(*mula bandha*)

diagram by: Alan Finger

How-to

On the inhalation, feel an electrical current of energy move from the base of the spine (*mula bandha*) up the front of the body, pass through the space between the collarbones, and continue to cross above the back of the head, to the top fontanel (*sahasrara* chakra) and lower into the middle of the brain (*ajna* chakra). This creates a "half figure-8" pathway up the front of the body.

On the exhalation, the awareness moves from the middle of the brain (*ajna* chakra) straight back to the C7 vertebra, which is the bump bone at the back of the neck, down the back passage of the body, past the tailbone, and back to the pelvic floor (*mula bandha*). This creates the second half of the figure-8 pathway down the back of the body.

Be sure to trace these movements of your awareness within the pacing of your breath. If you disconnect from your breath, you disconnect from your awareness and go outside your own healthy boundaries. *Arohan awarohan* is a profound technique that keeps us in our own truth, connected to our authentic self. You can integrate this *kriya* into any one of the poses. Use this technique in seated meditation to lead you back to *brahma nadi* and the state of pure consciousness.

THE PRACTICE

Here is a list of fifty-four poses, plus the Sun Salutations, that will help you to live in the light and build a foundation for a well-rounded, integrated, and embodied yoga practice. The poses are divided by category, but you only need to choose one or two poses from each class to create an empowered and inspiring practice. These postures cover all major muscle groups in the body, but, most importantly, you strengthen your muscle of self-study. Check in with your body every day and listen to the messages it is sending you: How is your energy feeling today? What does your body need? What will take you into a state of ease and lightness of being? Although consistency is required to reap the benefits of this practice, it is not always a linear process. Every day is different, so it is essential to focus on your internal space and not on the results. As Patanjali stated in sutra 2.14: "Practice becomes firmly grounded when well attended to for a long time, without break, and in all earnestness." Let the practice be the outcome. Once you understand the power of each asana, you can begin to use these poses as tools to reinvent your body, resurrect your soul, and live in the light that is your birthright.

SIMPLE STANDING POSES

The poses that fall under this category are stabilizing, neutralizing, and highly effective for creating steadiness in the legs, openness in the heart, and lightness in the mind. They are beneficial for beginners and therapeutic for anyone with balance issues or injuries that affect the knees, low back, shoulders, or neck.

MOUNTAIN POSE:
TADASANA

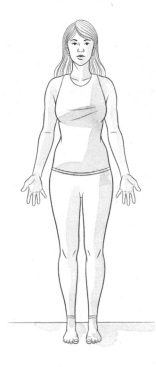

Overview: Tadasana is the foundation for all the other poses. Like a mountain, this pose is strong and steady. This pose helps us to embody stability through our feet and our legs. At the same time, we are also establishing a connection to the infinite intelligence of the universe through the crown chakra. When we understand our physical habits in *Tadasana*, we can see how they play out in all the other postures and life in general. To stand in *Tadasana* is to stand in our power, in our presence, in our own sovereign self.

How-to: Come to a standing position with your feet inner-hip distance apart and the heels behind the widest part of your feet. Now lift your toes off the floor, spread them apart, and lower them back down. Feel as if you could suction the Earth up through the soles of your feet so that you activate your quadriceps and lift the pelvic floor slightly. Firm your lower abdominal muscles slightly to support your lower back and feel the side ribs expanding with your breath. Now let your palms face forward and feel spaciousness across your collarbones. Allow your head and neck to float freely on top of your spine.

Benefits: Physically, *Tadasana* strengthens the ankles, legs, lower abdomen, buttocks, and back muscles. It tones the pelvic floor and aligns the spine for proper posture.

Energetically, *Tadasana* helps to create a balance between steadiness and ease. It brings us into *satva guna*, or homeostasis. When performed correctly, *Tadasana* balances all the chakras, but it is specifically helpful in balancing the first chakra. Engage *mula bandha*. Increases *apana vayu*.

Therapeutic applications: Relieves sciatica, helps with anxiety, corrects poor posture, and reduces flat feet.

Helpful tips: Depending on the width of your hips and the structure of your knees, you might need to move your feet a little wider to ensure that they align with your inner hips. You can also take a wider stance if you feel off-balance or use the wall or a chair for support. To strengthen *mula bandha*, place a block or cushion between your thighs (while standing in the posture).

UPWARD WORSHIP POSE:
URDHVA HASTASANA

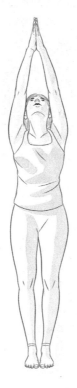

Overview: Upward Worship pose is the blueprint for many of the other chest openers that we practice in yoga. Bringing the palms to touch, we merge the dualities of right and left. By gazing toward the ceiling or the sky, we honor the infinite intelligence that is all around us.

How-to: From Mountain pose, inhale and lift the arms overhead, lengthening through the side and the back of your body. Extend through the elbows and fingertips as you bring the palms together.

Let your gaze lift slightly toward the thumbs, keeping the lower abdomen engaged and the back of the neck long.

Benefits: Physically, Upward Worship pose strengthens the legs, the lower abdomen, and the upper back. It stretches the belly, the rib cage, the chest, and the shoulders.

Energetically, Upward Worship pose helps us to shift our perspective. It is energizing and awakening, and can help elevate our mood. It activates the first, the fourth, and the fifth chakras.

Engage *mula bandha* and slight *uddiyana bandha*. Stimulates *prana vayu*.

Therapeutic applications: Helps with fatigue, asthma, and indigestion.

Helpful tips: If your shoulders are tight, bring your fingertips together to touch as you gaze up. You can also keep your arms shoulder-distance apart or slightly wider. If you have any neck issues, keep your gaze forward and your head in a neutral position.

CHAIR POSE:
UTKATASANA

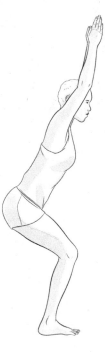

Overview: We often refer to *Utkatasana* as "Chair pose" when, in fact, the actual translation of the word from Sanskrit is "Fierce pose." This shape teaches us how to endure challenging situations with a sense of patience, tolerance, and curiosity, tapping into the truly powerful nature of our being, which is required for growth and transformation.

How-to: From *Tadasana*, walk the inner edges of your feet in to touch one another. Inhale, stretch your arms up alongside your ears, shoulder-distance apart, and extend through your fingertips. As you exhale, bend your knees, and allow your sit bones, or the lower area of your pelvis, to move back toward the wall behind you. At the same time, lift your hip bones away from your thighs and feel the engagement of your lower abdominal muscles. Keep the head and neck neutral and relax your jaw.

Benefits: Physically, Chair pose strengthens the ankles, the legs, the buttocks, the lower abdomen, the upper back, and the upper arms. It opens the chest and shoulders. Chair pose also stimulates the abdominal organs, the diaphragm, and the heart.

Energetically, Chair pose creates a strong sense of grounding and stability. It enables us to explore our tolerance for discomfort and how we respond to challenging situations. It activates the first chakra.

Engage *mula bandha* and slight *uddiyana bandha* to help lift *udana*. Stimulates *samana vayu*.

Therapeutic applications: Helps reduce flat feet; promotes the rehabilitation of ankle and knee injuries.

Helpful tips: If your shoulders are tight, keep the arms parallel to the floor, shoulder-distance apart. To help stabilize the legs, place a block in between the knees. If balance is an issue, practice this pose with your sacrum against the wall.

BLOWN PALM POSE:
PARSVA URDVA HASTASANA

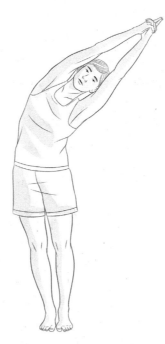

Overview: Blown Palm pose is a graceful embodiment of the palm tree, which can sway in the wind while remaining rooted at the base. This pose teaches us how to be flexible and fluid, yet steady and unwavering, to literally bend but not break.

How-to: From Mountain pose, stretch your arms overhead and bring your palms together to touch. Interlace your last three fingers and thumb, keeping your index fingers pointing straight up toward the ceiling. As you inhale, lengthen through the side body, and as you exhale, side-bend your torso over to your right, pressing into your left foot. Keep your abdominal muscles engaged to protect your lower back. Stay here and breathe, lengthening both sides of your waist evenly. On your next inhale, come back to center, keeping your arms overhead. As you next exhale, side-bend to your left, pressing into your right foot. Inhale and come back to center. On your exhale, lower both arms down alongside the body.

Benefits: Physically, Blown Palm pose opens the outer hips. It stretches the lower back, the waist, and the intercostal muscles between the ribs. It also opens the shoulders and tones the oblique abdominal muscles.

Energetically, Blown Palm pose opens the first and fourth chakras. This pose helps to stimulate the body's solar and lunar energy channels, known as *pingala* and *ida nadis*, located on the right and left sides of the body.

Engage *mula bandha* and slight *uddiyana bandha*. Stimulates *prana vayu*.

Therapeutic applications: Blown Palm pose helps with asthma and upper-respiratory congestion. It relieves sciatica and scoliosis and can reduce the effects of flat feet.

Helpful tips: If your shoulders are tight, hold on to the wrist of the opposite side from the one you are leaning toward. You can also keep one hand down alongside your body while the opposite arm reaches up and overhead, side-bending toward the side of the lowered arm.

STANDING HIP OPENERS

The greatest number of postures that we see in modern yoga fall under this category. When done correctly, these poses can simultaneously strengthen and stretch most of the major muscle groups in the body. These poses are most beneficial in building the muscles of the quadriceps, which helps to prevent conditions such as lower back pain and poor posture. The standing hip openers also teach us the qualities of balance, strength, empowerment, and perseverance.

LOW LUNGE POSE:
ANJANEYASANA

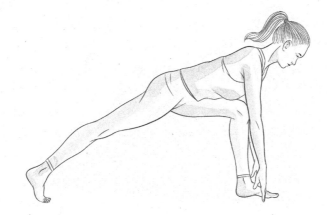

Overview: Low Lunge is sometimes called "runner's lunge" because it is the same position you'll see track runners take just before they are about to make a sprint. Overall, this pose is a safe and effective way to begin opening the iliopsoas muscle, which is the muscle that connects the lower body to the upper body. The muscle's primary function is to enable you to bend at the hip, and it's an integral part of our ability to stand, walk, and run.

How-to: From Standing Forward Bend, inhale and lengthen your chest forward, reaching toward the wall in front of you. As you next exhale, step the left foot back toward the back edge of your mat. Align your front knee directly over your ankle and press the back heel straight back toward the wall behind you. Keep your back thigh straight and strong. Draw the right hip back, so it's even with the left hip, and lengthen evenly through both sides of your torso. Reach through the center of your chest and keep the back of your neck long. Relax the tops of your shoulders and gaze toward a fixed point in front of you.

Benefits: Physically, Low Lunge both strengthens and stretches the quadriceps and the hip flexors. It tones the lower abdominal muscles and the muscles along the spine, and is a mild chest opener.

Energetically, Low Lunge is both grounding and releasing at the same time. It is a simple yet profound embodiment of *sthira* and *sukha*, which in Sanskrit mean "steadiness" and "ease." It opens the first and second chakras.

Engage *slight treta bandha.* Stimulates *samana vayu.* Engage *vajroli mudra* to create length in the back of the body.

Therapeutic applications: Can be helpful in relieving pain from sciatica and scoliosis, and may help with the rehabilitation of ankle and knee injuries.

Helpful tips: Lower the back knee down, either onto the mat or onto a blanket for a deeper stretch in the psoas. Use blocks underneath each hand to help lengthen the spine and open the chest.

WARRIOR 1 POSE:
VIRABHADRASANA 1

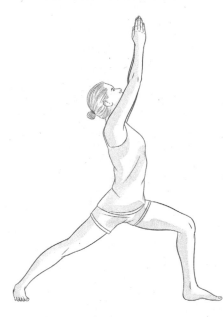

Overview: As the first of the three Warrior poses, Warrior 1 pose invokes the qualities one needs for battle: perseverance, strength, and commitment. In the case of the asanas, the battleground is not on a field, per se, but within the self. The strength we cultivate from the Warrior poses helps us break through our own limiting patterns to a state of freedom and transcendence.

How-to: From Low Lunge pose, place your back left heel flat on the floor, slightly left of center. Continue to root down into the back foot as you lift your torso into an upright position, drawing your left hip and left rib cage forward toward the front of your mat. Draw your navel back toward your spine and raise your arms overhead, lifting from the lower ribs toward your fingertips. Bring your palms together to touch and gaze toward the hands, keeping the back of your neck long.

Benefits: Physically, this pose strengthens the ankles, the legs, the arms, and the back, and stretches the Achilles tendons, the calves, and the hip flexors. It also opens the chest and the lungs.

Energetically, Warrior 1 pose helps to improve balance, focus, and concentration. It is grounding and increases the qualities of the earth element within us. It works on the first chakra.

Engage *mula bandha* and slight *uddiyana bandha*. Stimulates *prana vayu*. Engage *vajroli mudra* to create length in the back of the body.

Therapeutic applications: This pose is helpful in alleviating sciatica and lower back pain and can help ease asthma and indigestion symptoms.

Helpful tips: To allow more mobility in your pelvis, widen the distance between your feet and make your stance slightly shorter. If balance is an issue, anchor your back heel against the wall. If your shoulders are tight, keep the hands shoulder-distance apart or slightly wider.

WARRIOR 2 POSE:
VIRABHADRASANA 2

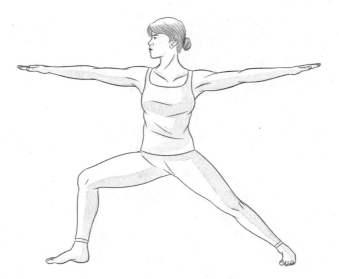

Overview: Warrior 2 pose is one of the most accessible of all the standing hip openers because it does not require too much range in the hips. As one of the three Warrior poses, the stance of Warrior 2 pose elicits a sense of security, strength, concentration, and will. It empowers us to take up the space we are in wholeheartedly.

How-to: From *Tadasana*, take your feet a little wider than leg's distance apart. Pivot your right foot forward toward the front of your mat; make sure the heel of the right foot aligns with the arch of your back foot. Now pivot your back toes in slightly so that the toes line up with the front left corner edge of your mat. Stretch your arms out in a "T" position, bringing your hands in line with your shoulders. Inhale, and gaze out over your right middle finger. As you exhale, bend the right knee and align it directly over the second and third toes. Keep maintaining a subtle lift through your pelvic floor. Relax the tops of your shoulders, soften your facial muscles, and let your *drishti*, or gaze, rest over the right middle finger. Breathe fluidly in and out.

Benefits: Physically, Warrior 2 pose strengthens the ankles, the knees, and the quadriceps. It also helps to tone the pelvic floor and stretches the groins, the chest, the lungs, and the shoulders.

Energetically, Warrior 2 pose builds endurance and patience, increases focus and concentration, and helps with balance. It strengthens the first and second chakras, helping improve stability, steadiness, and connection to the Earth. Simultaneously, it engages and opens our centers of creativity and sexuality.

Engage *mula bandha* and slight *uddiyana bandha*. Stimulates *apana vayu*.

Therapeutic applications: This pose can help relieve backache and improve the arches in the feet. It is also helpful for addressing infertility, osteoporosis, and sciatica.

Helpful tips: If balance is an issue, practice this pose with your back against the wall. If your hips are tight, pivot the back toes in even more, or adjust the space between the front and back foot so that your feet are heel to heel instead of heel to arch.

REVERSE WARRIOR POSE:
VIPARITA VIRABHADRASANA

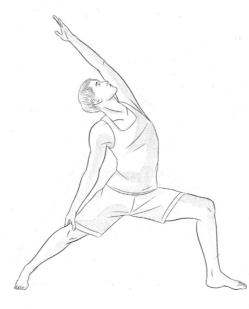

Overview: Often referred to as "peaceful warrior," Reverse Warrior pose brings a softer side to Warrior 2 pose. It opens the heart and lifts the gaze toward the sky, reminding us that we can be both strong and at peace simultaneously.

How-to: From Warrior 2 pose, spin the right palm to face the ceiling. On an inhale, lift through your torso and slide the back arm toward the back leg. At the same time, move the right arm up by the right ear. Engage your lower abdominal muscles and lengthen both sides of your waist evenly. On your next exhalation, come back to Warrior 2 pose.

Benefits: Physically, Reverse Warrior pose helps tone the lower abdomen and the side obliques. In addition to its strengthening effects on the quadriceps, this pose stretches the muscles along the lumbar spine. These are known as the "QL," or the quadratus lumborum. Reverse Warrior pose is an excellent pose to stretch the intercostal muscles, which help to free the breath. It opens the shoulders and the chest muscles.

Energetically, Reverse Warrior pose is stimulating because it moves the breath up into the upper chest. It encourages inhalation and engages the first, second, and fourth chakras, which induces feelings of love, compassion, and gratitude.

Engage *mula bandha*. Stimulates *prana vayu*.

Therapeutic applications: This pose can help relieve backache and improve the arches in the feet. It helps with asthma and upper-respiratory congestion.

Helpful tips: If balance is an issue, practice this pose with your back against the wall. To alleviate stress on your quadriceps, straighten your front leg. You can also practice this posture sitting on a chair.

SIDE ANGLE POSE:
PARSVAKONASANA

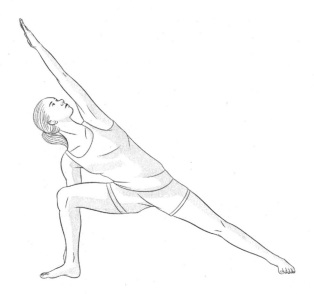

Overview: This full-body stretch and strength-building posture engages many of the major muscle groups, cultivating a sense of structure and expansion at the same time. It opens both the lower body, which represents our connection to the Earth, and the upper body, which represents our connection to pure intelligence.

How-to: From Warrior 2 pose, inhale and reach your right arm forward toward the front of your mat, lengthening your torso over your front thigh. On your exhale, lower the right hand down to the floor or place it on a block. Now spin the palm of your left hand forward toward the front of your mat and bring the top arm alongside your top ear. Keeping your front knee directly over your second and third toes, begin to rotate your top ribs toward the wall behind you, working to stack your rib cage. Breathe evenly into your front and back ribs. Shift your gaze up toward the top arm. Keep the same foot alignment as in *Virabhadrasana 2*.

Benefits: Physically, this pose strengthens the muscles of the legs and the ankles. It opens the groins and stretches the waist, the arms, the chest, the lower back, the intercostal muscles, and the lungs.

Energetically, Side Angle pose builds endurance and patience, increases focus and concentration, and helps with balance. It can help elevate your mood and combat mild depression. It works on the first chakra to help improve stability, steadiness, and connection to the Earth.

Engage *mula bandha* and slight *uddiyana bandha*. Stimulates *apana* and *udana vayu*.

Therapeutic applications: Helps alleviate constipation, infertility, sciatica, osteoporosis, and lower back pain.

Helpful tips: If balance is an issue, practice this pose with your back against the wall. To modify, rest your right forearm on your front thigh and raise the other arm overhead. Keep the top arm in line with your shoulder if your shoulders are tight, with fingertips pointing straight toward the ceiling. If you have any neck discomfort, keep your gaze forward toward the wall your torso is facing.

TRIANGLE POSE:
TRIKONASANA

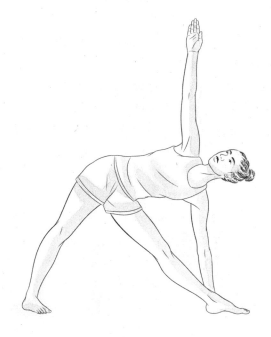

Overview: It is said that the triangle is the most stable of all the geometric shapes. It awakens us to the strong, dense power of the Earth that we can experience through our legs. Concurrently, we become more aware of the field of pure potential through the direction of the top arm.

How-to: From *Tadasana*, step or jump your legs wide, about a leg's distance apart, keeping your feet parallel. Pivot your right foot out at a 90-degree angle so that all five toes point toward the front of your mat. Pivot your back toes in at a 45-degree angle so that the toes point toward the left front corner edge of your mat. Inhale and lift your arms in a "T" position. On your exhale, bend at the right hip and reach your right arm toward the front of your mat. Lower your right hand down, either to your right shin or onto a block outside your right foot. Lift your left arm toward the ceiling. You can either gaze toward your top arm or, if that bothers your neck, gaze forward toward the wall in front of you.

Benefits: Physically, this pose opens the hamstrings, the hips, the groins, the chest, the shoulders, and the spine. It strengthens the ankles, the calves, the abdomen, the side obliques, and the upper back.

Energetically, *Trikonasana* is stimulating and increases focus and concentration. It activates the first, second, and fourth chakras.

Engage slight *mula bandha* to help reverse *apana vayu*. Engage slight *jalandhara bandha* to encourage energy movement to the crown. Stimulates *udana vayu*.

Therapeutic applications: Helps alleviate flat feet, infertility, neck pain, osteoporosis, and sciatica.

Helpful tips: If balance is an issue, practice this pose with your back against the wall. If your hamstrings are tight, place your hand on a block or a chair outside your front foot. If you have any neck sensitivity, fix your gaze forward or down toward your front foot.

HALF MOON POSE:
ARDHA CHANDRASANA

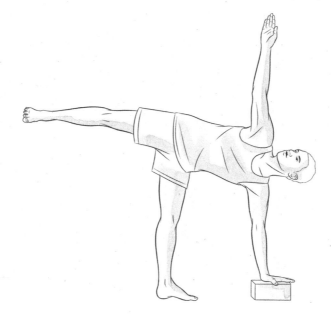

Overview: Like the moon, this pose teaches us about the significance of transition. How you enter into the pose will determine your ability to sustain the pose. When we get distracted or disconnected from our actions, we easily fall off-center. But when our actions are mindful, we can move through change without losing our connection to our innermost self.

How-to: From Triangle pose, place your left hand on your left hip and look down at your right foot. Bend your right knee and begin to slide your block or your hand forward about a foot. Now drag your back foot in and start to transfer your weight fully onto your right

foot. Pause. On your inhale, begin to straighten your right leg and lift
your left leg off the floor, pressing through the heel of the left foot as
if you were pushing it into a wall, so that the leg is straight and strong.
Stack your left rib cage on top of your right rib cage. Your left shoulder should align with the top of your right shoulder. Once you feel
steady, you can extend your left arm toward the ceiling and let your
gaze follow.

Benefits: Physically, this pose strengthens the ankles, the thighs,
the buttocks, the abdomen, and the spine. It stretches the groins, the
hamstrings and the calves, the shoulders, the chest, and the spine.

Energetically, Half Moon pose improves balance, focus, concentration, and coordination. It activates the first, second, and sixth
chakras.

Engage slight *mula bandha* and *uddiyana bandha* to help lift *apana
vayu*. Engage slight *jalandhara bandha* to encourage energy movement to the crown. Stimulates prana and *udana vayu*.

Therapeutic applications: Can relieve lower back pain when practiced against the wall, especially for pregnant women in their second
and third trimester.

Helpful tips: If balance is an issue, practice this pose with your
back against the wall. You can also start with the top hand on the top
hip and keep your gaze down toward the floor to maintain steadiness.
If your hamstrings are tight, place a block underneath your bottom
hand. As you did in the Triangle pose, fix your gaze forward or down
toward the front foot if you have any neck sensitivity.

LIZARD POSE:
UTTHAN PRISTHANA

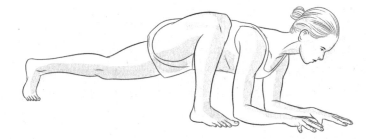

Overview: Lizard pose is one of the most effective poses to open the hips. By targeting the three main muscles of the hips—the hip flexors, the gluteal muscles, and the groins—it facilitates a profound release of the whole pelvic region on both a physical and an energetic level. This pose helps us to move through our emotions with compassion and courage.

How-to: From Low Lunge, lower your back knee down onto the floor or onto a blanket for support. Walk your right foot toward the right edge of your mat and point the toes out slightly toward the corner. Be sure to keep the right knee directly over the right ankle. Place your hands on the inside of the right foot. Either stay here or lower your elbows to the floor for a deeper stretch. You can keep the back knee down for a more passive stretch or lift the back knee off the floor for a more active version of the pose.

Benefits: Physically, this pose opens the quadriceps, the hip flexors, the hamstrings, the groins, and the gluteal muscles. It strengthens the quadriceps and the lower abdominal muscles. It also helps to open the shoulders and the chest.

Energetically, Lizard pose promotes our ability to be flexible—not just in our bodies but in our lives. This pose works on the second chakra, which is the element of water, and water governs our polarities. It is responsible for our ability to be fluid in life and to "go with the flow," so this shape opens that part of our consciousness. The hips also tend to hold a lot of unprocessed emotions; therefore, Lizard pose helps to release memories, feelings, and beliefs that get lodged in this area and that keep us from recognizing our essential nature.

Engage *mula bandha* to help reverse *apana vayu.* Engage *vajroli mudra.* Stimulates *vyana vayu.*

Therapeutic applications: Can help relieve lower back pain, increase fertility, and alleviate menstrual discomfort. Lizard pose is also helpful for women who are pregnant.

Helpful tips: Keep the back knee on the floor for a more receptive version of this pose. If your hips are tight, place a block underneath each forearm, so you maintain space in the chest and shoulders.

GARLAND POSE:
MALASANA

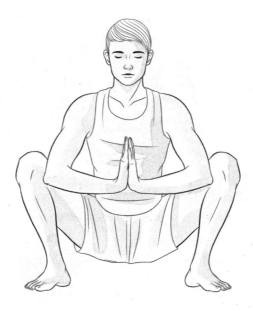

Overview: This hip opener can either be restful or highly challenging depending on your anatomy. The pose gets its name from the small round gems that make up a *mala*, a sacred string of beads used for chanting or praying in India. Creating this shape with our own body reminds us that asana is its own form of prayer.

How-to: From Mountain pose, take your legs as wide as your mat or slightly wider than the distance of your hips. Bend at your knees and begin to lower your sit bones down toward the floor. If your heels start to lift off the floor, pause and breathe there. Bring your palms together to touch. If your knees are completely bent, take your elbows to your inner thighs to help open the hips and press the palms of your hands firmly together to help broaden across the sternum.

Benefits: Physically, Garland pose stretches the Achilles tendon, the groins, the gluteal muscles, and the torso. It also helps to open the chest and shoulders.

Energetically, Garland pose activates the first and second chakras and can be specifically helpful in stimulating sexual energy.

Engage a slight *mula bandha* to help balance that downward energy with an upward lift of the spine. There is a slight *jalandhara bandha* to keep the energy line from base to midbrain. Garland pose helps facilitate the movement of *apana* to ease elimination.

Therapeutic applications: Aids in digestion, relieves lower back pain, and is excellent for pregnant women to help with childbirth.

Helpful tips: If your ankle flexion is limited, place a folded blanket underneath your heels. If your knees cannot come into full flexion, place a block or two blocks underneath your sit bones. Place a block or a thick book between the palms to help broaden across the collarbones and draw the shoulder blades toward one another. If you have any knee or hip injuries, try this pose on your back with your hips close to a wall, your knees bent, your legs wide apart, and your feet pressing into the wall.

STANDING FORWARD BENDS

Standing forward bends are extremely useful both for increasing our physical range and decreasing our mental chatter. Anatomically, they open the hamstring muscles, which are the group of muscles responsible for much of our daily activities, such as walking, running, and climbing stairs. Energetically, the backs of the legs are where we store our unconscious patterning, the limiting beliefs and false narratives that we acquire from a very young age. Forward bends also encourage a deep sense of calm and letting go by gently lifting the diaphragm and facilitating the exhalation. Lastly, standing forward bends are a great lesson in the law of least effort. The more you soften in almost all these postures, the easier it is to come into the pose.

WIDE-LEGGED FORWARD BEND, VARIATION A:
PRASARITA PADDOTTANASANA

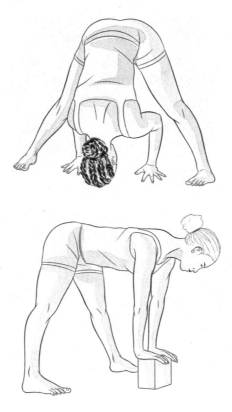

Overview: Wide-Legged Forward Bend A is an accessible yet profound way to stretch the hamstrings and maintain a sense of balance at your base. The symmetry and wide stance of the legs make this pose friendlier for those with tight hamstrings.

How-to: From Mountain pose, step or jump your legs wide to about a leg's distance apart. Keep all ten toes pointing forward and align the outer edges of your feet with the edges of the mat. Place your hands on your hips. Firm your quadriceps by suctioning the floor up through the soles of your feet. Inhale and lift your sternum toward the ceiling, keeping your lower belly engaged. As you exhale, hinge at your hips, and lower the torso down toward the floor. If your hands reach the mat, walk the fingertips back to line up with the toe tips. Spread your fingers wide and place the palms of the hands flat on the floor. Bend your elbows straight back toward the wall behind you and allow the crown of the head to move toward the mat. If the hands don't touch the floor, place a block underneath each hand.

Benefits: Physically, this pose stretches the hamstrings and the back. It strengthens the ankles and the front of the legs. It creates traction through the spine and can help to release the neck. It also stimulates the digestive process by directing circulation to the abdominal organs.

Energetically, Wide-Legged Forward Bend A helps unlock the unconscious, limiting beliefs stored in the backs of the legs. It helps relieve anxiety and frees up the exhalation, encouraging a sense of letting go. This pose can also shift our mental outlook, and it works on the first, sixth, and seventh chakras.

Engage *uddiyana* and *jalandhara bandha* to facilitate the movement of energy up to the crown. Engage *ashvini mudra* to create length in the spine. Stimulates *apana vayu*.

Therapeutic applications: Helps to relieve mild headaches and fatigue, and can alleviate mild backache.

Helpful tips: If your hamstrings are tight and your hands don't reach the floor, you can either place your hands on a chair or on blocks directly underneath your shoulders. For a more restorative

option, place a bolster or a block underneath your forehead. Reach
your arms out toward the wall opposite you, supporting yourself on
your fingertips and releasing your chest toward the floor.

Variation: For the added benefit of opening the shoulders, try this
same posture with your fingers interlaced behind you at the small of
your back. Draw your shoulder blades in toward one another and
press the palms of your hands together. Inhale and lift your sternum
toward the ceiling, keeping your lower belly engaged. As you exhale,
hinge at your hips, and lower the torso toward the floor, lifting your
arms away from your lower back. If your shoulders are tight, use a
strap in between the hands instead of interlacing the fingers.

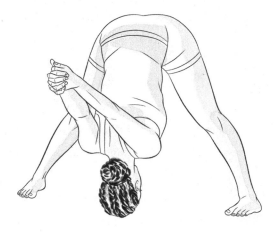

HALF-FORWARD BEND POSE:
ARDHA UTTANASANA

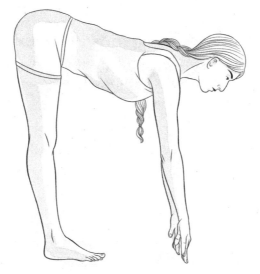

Overview: Often referred to as "Prepare pose," this asana "prepares" us to step back to Plank, jump back to Low Push-Up, and fold forward over the legs with a long spine and an open heart.

How-to: From intense stretch pose, inhale and slide your fingertips onto the floor, directly underneath your shoulders, and reach the center of the chest forward. Gaze forward to the front edge of your mat. Release the shoulder blades down, away from the ears, and keep the back of your neck long.

Benefits: Physically, Half-Forward Bend pose strengthens the legs, the abdominal muscles, the muscles along the spine, and the back of the neck. It stretches the hamstrings and opens the chest and shoulders.

Energetically, this pose increases focus. It works on the first and third chakras, cultivating both strength and flexibility at the same time.

Engage *mula bandha* and *jalandhara bandha*. Engage *ashvini mudra* to lengthen the spine. Stimulates *udana vayu*.

Therapeutic applications: Helps relieve lower back pain and hamstring injuries, and it's useful for pregnant practitioners.

Helpful tip: If your hamstrings are tight, either bend your knees or place a block underneath each hand.

INTENSE STRETCH POSE:
UTTANASANA

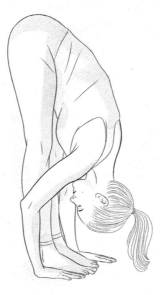

Overview: Intense Stretch pose is true to its name; it is a pose that is an intense release for the entire back of the body. This pose is usually offered as part of a more extensive sequence of postures, as in Sun Salutations. When it is held for long periods of time, it creates a profound sense of release in the physical, mental, and energetic layers of your being.

How-to: From Mountain pose, place your hands on your hips. Inhale and lift your sternum toward the ceiling, keeping your lower belly engaged. As you exhale, hinge at your hips, and lower the torso down toward the floor. If your hands do not reach the floor, bend your knees, or place blocks underneath each hand.

Benefits: Physically, Intense Stretch pose stretches the calves, the hamstrings, the hips, and the back. It strengthens the ankles and the quadriceps. The pose helps to create traction in the spine. Intense Stretch pose stimulates the digestive process by directing circulation to the abdominal organs. It also acts as a mild inversion, bringing blood to the brain and oxygenating your body's cells.

Energetically, Intense Stretch pose facilitates a sense of letting go by lifting the diaphragm up, which encourages the exhalation. It opens the back gates of all chakras, pacifying their rajasic qualities and increasing *tamas*—the quality of inertia. *Uttanasana* is also energetically cooling and can help us to see things from a new perspective.

Engage *mula*, *uddiyana*, and *jalandhara bandha* to facilitate the movement of energy up to the crown. Engage *ashvini mudra* to create length in the spine. Stimulates *apana vayu*.

Therapeutic applications: Intense Stretch pose is helpful for people with osteoporosis and sinusitis. It alleviates anxiety, fatigue, and headaches.

Helpful tips: Bend your knees or use blocks underneath each hand if your hamstrings are tight. Hold on to the opposite forearm with each hand and let your head and neck release toward the floor to make this pose more energetically passive.

SUN SALUTATION VARIATIONS

The Sun Salutation is a full-body warm-up and prayer to the sun. By practicing Sun Salute variations, we practice the art of *vinyasa*, which involves linking each breath with movement. We invigorate the body by initiating each posture from breath, build cardiovascular endurance, increase our fluidity, and create a moving meditation to anchor our mind.

SUN BREATH:
SURYA PRANA

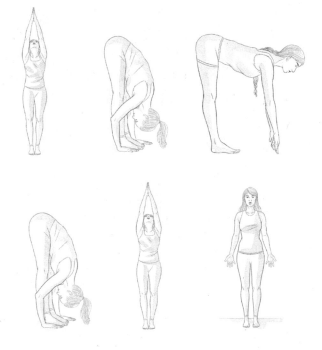

Overview: The Sun Breath series is a helpful place to begin learning Sun Salutations for the first time. It facilitates the benefits of connecting breath and movement without putting any strain on the joints. It is safe for anyone with wrist or shoulder injuries or those who want to moderately build heat in the body without too much intensity.

How-to: From *Tadasana*, follow each step, one breath per movement.

Inhale: Upward Worship pose

Exhale: Intense Stretch pose

Inhale: Half-Forward Bend pose

Exhale: Intense Stretch pose

Inhale: Upward Worship pose

Exhale: Mountain pose

Benefits: Physically, the Sun Breath series opens the shoulders, the chest cavity, and the hamstrings. It strengthens the muscles along the spine as well as the lower abdomen.

Energetically, this series is energizing, stimulating, and uplifting. It works on all the chakras and balances opposing forces, such as moving up and moving down, breathing in and breathing out, opening the front and opening the back of the body, which also opens each chakra's front and rear gates.

Engage *vajroli mudra* for *Urdva Hastasana*; *ashvini mudra* for *Uttanasana* and *Ardha Uttanasana*. Refer to individual poses for *bandhas*. Stimulates *vyana vayu*.

Therapeutic applications: The Sun Breath series can help reduce anxiety and restlessness.

Helpful tips: Place a block underneath each hand for the forward bends. Bend the knees if you have any lower back issues. If the shoulders are tight, keep the hands shoulder-distance apart in Upward Worship pose.

SUN SALUTATION A:
SURYA NAMASKAR A

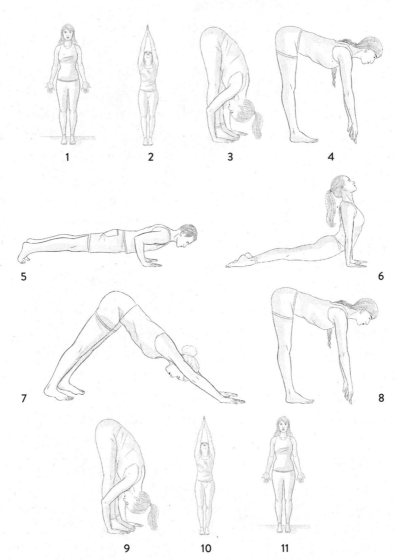

Overview: There are traditionally eleven poses linked together that make up the Sun Salutation A sequence. The series is a full-body warm-up that works on the dualities of right and left, up and down, inhalation and exhalation, strength and flexibility, and expansion and contraction. Through the practice of Sun Salutations, we invoke the qualities of the sun that are within us all: heat, radiance, energy, light, and magnetism.

How-to: From Mountain pose, follow each step, using one breath per movement:

Inhale: Upward Worship pose
Exhale: Intense Stretch pose
Inhale: Half-Forward Bend pose
Exhale: Low Push-Up pose
Inhale: Upward-Facing Dog pose
Exhale: Downward-Facing Dog pose
Inhale: Gaze up to your hands
Exhale: Step or jump your feet to your hands
Inhale: Half-Forward Bend pose
Exhale: Intense Stretch pose
Inhale: Upward Worship pose
Exhale: Mountain pose

Benefits: Physically, Sun Salutation A aids in cardiovascular health by increasing blood flow throughout the body. Like the Sun Breath, this sequence of postures is energizing, awakening, and heat building. It strengthens the muscles in the legs, the abdomen, the upper body, and the back. It also opens the hamstrings, the quadriceps, the upper back, and the chest.

Energetically, Sun Salutation A enables us to embody the qualities of the sun: warmth, energy, radiance and *tejas*, the magnetism that is created by the essence of fire. It works on all the chakras, especially the third and fourth chakras. There is a harmonizing effect that comes from stretching and strengthening the muscles and opening the front and back of the body, bringing us into *satva guna*. When done rhythmically on the breath, Sun Salutation A can induce the benefits of a moving meditation, which include slowing down the mind, slowing down the brain waves, and calming restlessness or agitation.

Engage *vajroli mudra* for *urdva hastasana* and *Urdva Mukha Svanasana*; *ashvini mudra* for *Uttanasana*, *Ardha Uttanasana*, and *Adho Mukha Svanasana*. Refer to individual poses for *bandhas*. Engage *mula bandha* when jumping forward or backward. Works on *samana* and *vyana vayu*.

Therapeutic applications: Sun Salutation A can help lower blood sugar levels, balance the hormones, and aid in countering obesity.

Helpful tips: Since this series involves many poses linked together, it could be useful to take pauses in between each posture if you are new to the practice. If the hips sink in Plank pose or Low Push-Up pose, lower the knees to the floor to support the lower belly and maintain a long spine. If you have any wrist or lower back sensitivity, practice Baby Cobra pose (see page 224) instead of Upward-Facing Dog. Try practicing up to five series in a row to build endurance.

STANDING TWISTS

Twisting postures have the unique ability to bring us up against our own limitations. They teach us how to find freedom in challenging circumstances and recruit the breath as a form of leverage. Since twists work on the third chakra, they aid in the digestion of our food, and the processing of thoughts and emotions. In addition to being detoxifying, twists facilitate a long and healthy spine.

TWISTING CHAIR POSE:
PARIVRITTA UTKATASANA

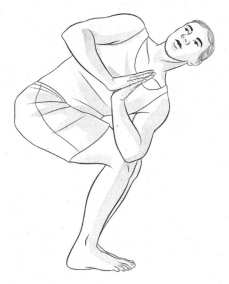

Overview: This dynamic, heat-building pose teaches us how to stay rooted and fluid simultaneously.

How-to: From Chair pose, bring your palms together, touching, at the center of your chest. Breathe in and lift your sternum away from your pelvis. Breathe out and twist to the right, hooking your left upper arm to your outer right thigh. As you inhale, lengthen your spine and as you exhale, rotate around the axis of your spine. Keep your shoulder blades moving away from your ears and broaden across your collarbones.

Benefits: Physically, Twisting Chair pose strengthens the ankles, the quadriceps, the buttocks, and the abdomen. It tones the digestive organs and the kidneys, facilitating the detoxification process. Spinal rotation compresses the intervertebral discs, which expand like a sponge when coming out of the twist. As a result, Twisting Chair pose helps to lengthen the spine.

Energetically, Twisting Chair pose activates the first and third chakras, stimulating heat, transformation, and empowerment while also offering the benefits of stability and structure. This pose increases *agni*, the digestive fire responsible for converting matter into waste. It also increases *tapas*, the quality of heat that creates discipline, patience, and ultimate transformation.

Engage *mula bandha* and *uddiyana bandha*. Increases *samana vayu*.

Therapeutic applications: Great for alleviating scoliosis, restless mind, and sluggish metabolism.

Helpful tips: If you feel restricted in the twist, place the left hand to the outside of the right thigh. Move your right hand onto the sacrum, allowing the twist to happen in the middle of the spine. Place a block in between the thighs to keep the knees aligned. Not indicated for pregnant women.

TWISTING SIDE ANGLE POSE:
PARIVRITTA PARSVAKONASANA

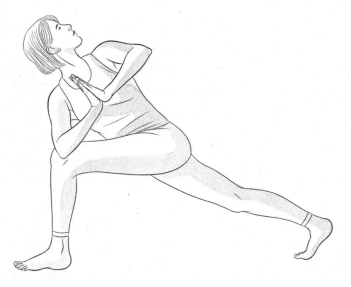

Overview: This pose teaches the qualities of perseverance, patience, groundedness, and flexibility all at the same time. It can be a great introductory pose for learning the actions of twists in a step-by-step process.

How-to: From Low Lunge, inhale and lift the arms overhead. On the exhale, lengthen your torso over the front thigh, keeping your arms by the ears. Bring your palms together to touch at the center of the chest. Rotate your left upper arm to the outside of the right outer thigh. As you breathe in, lift the sternum, and as you breathe out, rotate around the axis of the spine, keeping your back thigh straight and strong.

Benefits: Physically, Twisting Side Angle pose strengthens the ankles, the quadriceps, the buttocks, and the abdomen. It also stretches the quadriceps, the hip flexors, and the gluteal muscles. It helps to improve balance. See Twisting Chair pose (page 190) for the digestive and spinal benefits of this pose.

The energetic benefits of this posture are very similar to those of Twisting Chair pose: It activates the first and third chakras, stimulating heat, transformation, and empowerment while also offering the benefits of stability and structure.

Engage *mula bandha* and *uddiyana bandha.* Increases *samana vayu.*

Therapeutic applications: Great for alleviating the discomfort of scoliosis by twisting away from the contracted side of the body. Focuses a distracted mind and stimulates a sluggish metabolism.

Helpful tips: If balance is an issue or you are not quite ready to practice this posture in its full expression, keep the back knee on the floor as you come into the twist. For a deeper expression of this pose, extend the bottom hand down toward the floor or place it on a block. Extend the top arm toward the ceiling. Not indicated for pregnant women.

TWISTING TRIANGLE POSE:
PARIVRITTA TRIKONASANA

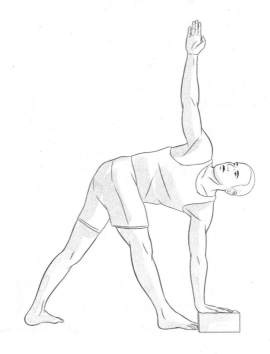

Overview: The Twisting Triangle pose is a multipurpose pose because it targets so many different areas of the body. It teaches us how to remain committed to the process while surrendering the results. This concept is known in Sanskrit as *abhyasa and vairagya* (sutra 1.13–1.14).

How-to: From Mountain pose, step your left foot back about 3 feet behind you. Keep a centerline between the front and back foot so that your feet are not on a "tightrope." Place the right hand on your right hip and extend the left arm up by the left ear, pointing the fingertips toward the ceiling. Inhale, and lengthen the spine. As you exhale, bend at your hips and extend your left arm over the front leg, lowering the left hand to the outside of your right foot. Rotate your right rib cage on top of your left rib cage and stack your right shoulder on top of your left shoulder, shifting your gaze toward the extended top arm.

Benefits: Physically, Twisting Triangle pose opens the hamstrings, the hips, and the shoulders. It strengthens the abdomen and the upper back. See Twisting Chair pose (page 190) for the digestive and spinal benefits.

Energetically, Twisting Triangle pose activates the first and third chakras. It simultaneously releases the unconscious beliefs that get lodged in the backs of the legs and develops the heat necessary to break them down. In addition to the heat-building benefits generated by the other standing twists, this pose creates a sense of balance and release at the same time.

Engage *mula bandha* and *uddiyana bandha.* Increases *samana vayu.*

Therapeutic applications: See Twisting Side Angle pose (page 192).

Helpful tips: If your hamstrings are tight, place a block underneath the bottom hand. If your shoulders are tight, place the top hand on the sacrum instead of extending it toward the ceiling. If you feel restricted in the twist, place the block on the inside of the front foot instead of on the outside.

BALANCING POSES

Standing on one leg requires not only focus and concentration but also patience and humility. The ancient *rishis* practiced standing on one leg as a way to build *tapas*, the austerity that helps us break through the mind's limitations. It is hard for us to plan our day or think about something that happened in the past when we are standing on one leg. In addition to learning how to be in the "now," balancing poses offer us the gift of humbleness, learning how to be with our own frustration when things don't always work out as planned.

TREE POSE:
VRIKSHASANA

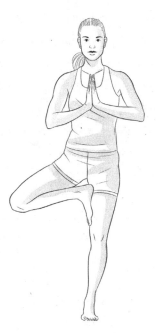

Overview: Tree pose is a simple yet powerful pose that trains us to get out of our minds and into the present moment. Just like its namesake, Tree pose teaches us how to root and rise at the same time. It empowers us to stay connected to one point of focus even if we're surrounded by distraction and chaos.

How-to: From Mountain pose, gaze on a point a little bit in front of you, preferably at something not moving. Shift your weight over to the left foot and lift the right heel off the floor. Keep drawing your outer left hip in toward the midline as you lift the right foot off the floor, and rotate your right thighbone open toward the right. Place your right foot to the inside of the left thigh. Bring your palms to touch at the center of the chest or lift your arms overhead in a "V" shape.

Benefits: Physically, Tree pose strengthens the ankles, the knees, and the thighs, and tones the pelvic floor. It opens the inner and outer hips and helps to lengthen the spine.

Energetically, Tree pose increases focus and concentration. It works on the first and sixth chakras, enabling us to get grounded in the legs and feet while developing *drishti*, focusing the gaze or direction of our eyes on a single point. Because our eyes reflect the activity of the mind, a steady gaze allows us to steady the mind. Tree pose can also help reduce anxiety or restlessness.

Engage *mula bandha.* Stimulates *apana vayu.*

Therapeutic applications: Helps with flat feet, osteoporosis, and anxiety. Can help alleviate the pain of sciatica.

Helpful tips: If your balance is precarious, start by placing the right foot either on the ankle or shin, avoiding the knee. You can also try this pose next to a wall or behind a chair to help maintain your balance.

LORD OF THE DANCER POSE:
NATARAJASANA

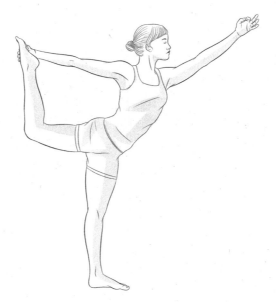

Overview: Nataraj is another name for Shiva, the deity of destruction. This pose symbolizes the cosmic dance of Shiva, who is the archetype of universal intelligence. Just as there is a dance of life and creativity, there is a dance of renunciation and letting go. When we honor that dance of destruction, we can consciously create anew.

How-to: From Mountain pose, shift your weight onto your left foot and bend your right leg straight back behind you. Take hold of the right foot or ankle with the right hand and extend your left arm straight out in front of you. Keep your eyes focused on one point as you begin to press your right foot into your right hand and your right hand into your right foot, lifting the foot away from your right buttock. Keep directing your right inner thigh toward the wall behind you as your lift your leg away from your body. Stay here and breathe for as long as you comfortably can.

Benefits: Physically, this posture stretches the hip flexors, the quadriceps, the chest, and the shoulders. It strengthens the ankles, the knees, and the thighs, and helps tone the lower abdominal muscles. This pose helps to improve balance and posture.

Energetically, Lord of the Dancer pose builds focus and concentration. It stretches the intercostal muscles, which serve to free up the breath. This pose also works on the first and fourth chakras, generating stability and fostering a sense of connection and emotional sensitivity. Stimulates *prana vayu.*

Therapeutic applications: Aids in digestion and relieves the pain of flat feet.

Helpful tips: To help with balance, use a wall or a chair to support the extended arm. If your quadriceps are tight, stay in an upright position and keep the foot of the bent leg closer to the buttocks.

EXTENDED HAND TO BIG TOE POSE:
UTTHITA HASTA PADANGUSTASANA

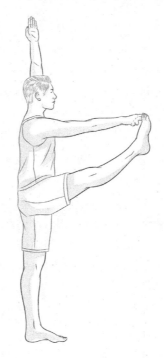

Overview: Although the traditional version of this pose is not recommended for beginners, there are many different versions of the
pose you can adapt to your own level. Like any situation in life, if we
get too far ahead of ourselves in this pose, we will get thrown off balance. By maintaining a slow and steady pace, we can stay present to
the quiet, still space within and be guided by it.

How-to: From Mountain pose, shift your weight over to the left
foot and draw your right knee in toward your chest. Grab hold of the
right big toe with the first two fingers of the right hand ("yogic toe

lock") and plug the right arm bone into the shoulder socket. Keep your right hip level with the left hip. Place your left hand on your left hip and keep your eyes steady on one point as you begin to extend the right leg forward, away from your right hip. Press into the ball of the right foot and spread the toes. Stay here or extend the left arm overhead. If you feel steady here, you can make the second variation by rolling the right thigh open to the right and extending the left arm out to the left.

Benefits: Physically, this pose strengthens the ankles, the knees, the quadriceps, the hip flexors, the abdomen, and the back. It opens the hamstrings and groins. It helps to improve balance.

Energetically, Extended Hand to Big Toe pose builds focus and concentration. It teaches the qualities of *sthira* and *sukha*, or "steadiness" and "ease," as referenced in the *Yoga Sutras of Patanjali* (sutra 2.46). It works on the first, second, and sixth chakras.

Engage *mula bandha* to reverse *apana* and increase *udana vayu.*

Therapeutic applications: Helps with flat feet, reduces anxiety, and relieves lower back pain.

Helpful tips: If your hamstrings are tight, use a strap or a towel to wrap around the sole of the foot of the extended leg. You can also rest your foot on a chair, at hip height or slightly lower, to help with balance or tight hamstrings. For a more dynamic experience in the extended leg and to create more spaciousness in the pelvis, place the extended leg's foot on the wall at hip height and press all four corners of the foot into the wall.

WARRIOR 3:
VIRABHADRASANA 3

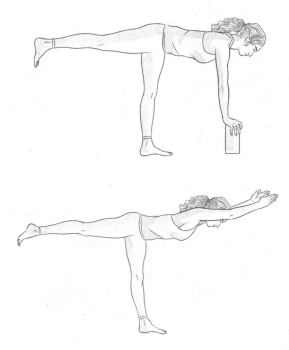

Overview: This Warrior pose is the most complex of the three. A great level of commitment and perseverance is required to sustain this pose, leaving us with the fruits of inner strength, will, and resilience.

How-to: From Warrior 1 pose, lengthen your torso forward over your front right leg and come onto the ball of the back foot. Transfer your weight completely onto your right foot as you lift the left foot off the floor, eventually bringing the foot in line with the pelvis. Press the sole of the left foot back toward the wall behind you. Angle the center of the chest forward toward the wall in front of you. Keep your hips level. Extend your arms out in front of you or to the side in a "T" position.

Benefits: Physically, this pose strengthens the ankles, the knees, the quadriceps, the abdomen, and the back. It also strengthens the upper body.

Energetically, Warrior 3 pose improves focus, concentration, will, and determination. It increases *tapas* and works on the first, third, and sixth chakras.

Engage *mula, uddiyana,* and slight *jalandhara bandha.* Stimulates *samana vayu.*

Therapeutic applications: This pose helps with flat feet, reduces anxiety, and improves posture. It can also be helpful in reducing lower back pain.

Helpful tips: If your hamstrings are tight or balance is an issue, place a block under each hand, directly underneath each shoulder. To help align and activate the back leg, place the foot on a wall or rest it on a chair at hip height.

EAGLE POSE:
GARUDASANA

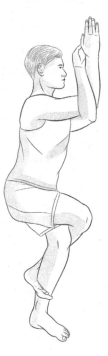

Overview: Although the Sanskrit meaning of this pose is translated as "eagle" in English, the *garuda* is a mythical, bird-like creature, the mount or vehicle (*vahana*) of Lord Vishnu, the archetype of sustainability. This pose teaches us about our ability to sustain and remain grounded in times of challenge or adversity.

How-to: From Chair pose, bring your hands to your hips and shift your weight over the left foot, extending the right leg out to the side. Keep your eyes steady on one point as you cross the right leg over the left leg, either resting the right foot against the left leg or hooking it around the left ankle. Stretch your arms wide in a "T" position and then bend your right elbow in so that your face is in line with your right palm. Now wrap the left arm underneath the right elbow. Then bring the backs of the hands to touch or the palms to touch. Stay here or begin to fold forward at your hips. Move your elbows in front of your knees and allow your shoulder blades to move away from one another. To come out of this pose, continue to hug your inner thighs toward one another, engage your lower abdomen, and use your gaze to help you to lift back up to an upright position.

Benefits: Physically, Eagle pose strengthens the ankles, the calves, the knees, the quadriceps, the inner thighs, and the abdomen. It stretches the gluteal muscles, the shoulders, and the muscles between the shoulder blades, known as the rhomboids.

Energetically, this pose improves focus, concentration, will, and perseverance. It increases *agni* and works on the first, third, fourth, and sixth chakras, and it opens the back gate of all the chakras when we practice the forward bend variation.

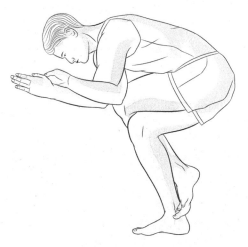

Engage *mula, uddiyana,* and *jalandhara bandha.* Stimulates *samana vayu.*

Therapeutic applications: Helps with flat feet and sciatica, reduces lower back pain, alleviates asthma and congestion in the lungs, and aids digestion.

Helpful tips: Depending on the anatomy of your body, you may or may not be able to hook the standing foot. As an alternative, rest the right foot on a block underneath the toes. If your shoulders are tight, hold on to a towel in between your hands. You can also try this pose with your seat against a wall to help with any balancing issues.

FOUR-LIMBED POSES

As bipeds, we are not accustomed to spending much time on our hands and knees or our hands and feet, but there are significant benefits to reorienting our relationship to the floor. This group of poses evokes the playfulness of our inner child and the stealth of our quadruped ancestors while also providing lower back relief.

COW POSE:
BITILASANA

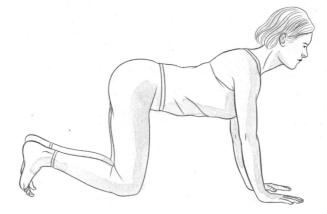

Overview: This gentle and therapeutic stretch is beneficial for most people, especially those who are pregnant or suffering from lower back pain. It taps into a sense of playfulness and ease. Usually, this posture is done in tandem with Cat pose (see page 212).

How-to: From hands and knees, align your wrists under your shoulders and your knees under your hips. Spread your fingers comfortably wide and press into the pads of your hands. As you inhale, reach the center of your chest forward, lifting your gaze and your sit bones up. Keep your shoulder blades away from your ears and the back of your neck long.

Benefits: Physically, Cow pose strengthens the muscles along the spine and the lower abdominal muscles. It stretches the wrists and strengthens the hands, the forearms, and the upper body. It adds mobility to the spine and gently stretches the torso and the front of the neck.

Energetically, this pose activates the inhalation, which is inspiring and energizing. It stimulates the fourth chakra and opens the whole front of the body, encouraging a sense of extroversion and connection to others.

Engage slight *mula bandha* to reverse the flow of *apana*; increases *prana vayu*. Engage *vajroli mudra* to create length in the back of the body.

Therapeutic applications: Excellent for pregnant women to help create space in the belly and relieve lower back discomfort; helps with mild scoliosis, corrects poor posture (kyphosis), and stimulates the liver and kidneys.

Helpful tips: This pose is usually done in tandem with Cat pose (see page 212), which creates a gentle and fluid moving meditation. Cow pose is an excellent introduction to *vinyasa*, or conscious movement on the breath. If your kneecaps are sensitive, place a folded blanket under your knees. If you have any wrist sensitivity, try this on your forearms or with a wedge underneath your hands. If you are using a wedge, place the highest part of the wedge under the heel of the hand and the lowest part of the wedge underneath your fingers.

CAT POSE:
MARJARYASANA

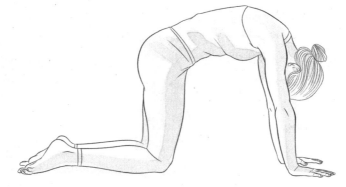

Overview: Like its counterpart, Cow pose, Cat pose is a simple and appropriate posture for almost any practitioner. As its name implies, this pose evokes our furtive, cat-like nature by gracefully stretching the whole back of the body and bringing our focus inward.

How-to: From hands and knees, align your wrists under your shoulders and your knees under your hips. Spread your fingers comfortably wide and press into the pads of your hands. Take a breath in, and as you exhale, draw the navel toward the spine, rounding your upper back and tucking in your tailbone. Let your head drop down toward the floor and stretch in between the shoulder blades.

Benefits: Physically, Cat pose stretches the muscles along the spine, the rhomboids, and the back of the neck. It stretches the wrists and strengthens the hands, the forearms, and the upper body. It improves digestion by massaging the digestive organs.

Energetically, this pose activates the exhalation, which is calming and soothing. It opens the back gates of all the chakras, especially the second, third, fourth, and fifth, inducing a state of introspection and connection inward.

Engage *mula, uddiyana,* and *jalandhara bandha,* or *treta bandha.* Increases *samana vayu.*

Therapeutic applications: Excellent for pregnant women to help create space in the belly and relieve lower back discomfort; helps with mild scoliosis, corrects poor posture (lordosis, or excessive inward curvature of the spine), helps with constipation.

Helpful tip: This pose is usually done in tandem with Cow pose (see page 210). Inhale: Cow. Exhale: Cat.

TIGER POSE:
VYAGHRASANA

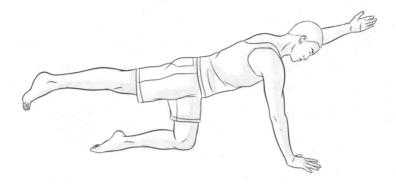

Overview: Like a tiger waking up from a nap, this pose stretches the opposing limbs of the body. It helps build symmetry in the body and dexterity in the mind, keeping us balanced, steady, and alert.

How-to: From hands and knees, stretch the right leg back at hip height, keeping all five toes pointing down toward the floor. Extend your left arm forward alongside your ear with your fingertips pointing toward the wall in front of you. Draw your navel toward the spine and gaze at a point a little bit in front of you. Breathe fully in and out.

Benefits: Physically, this pose strengthens the hamstrings, the gluteus muscles, the abdominal muscles, and the muscles along the spine. It helps to create symmetry in the body and works both hemispheres of the brain simultaneously.

Energetically, Tiger pose builds focus, concentration, and patience. It works on the third and sixth chakras.

Engage slight *mula bandha*, *uddiyana bandha*, and *jalandhara bandha*. Stimulates *samana vayu*.

Therapeutic applications: Excellent for pregnant women, eases the pain of scoliosis, reduces lower back pain, alleviates anxiety, stimulates digestion.

Helpful tips: If your kneecaps are sensitive, place a blanket underneath your knees. If your shoulders are tight, take the extended arm farther away from the ear or bend the elbow in a cactus position.

DOWNWARD-FACING DOG POSE:
ADHO MUKHA SVANASANA

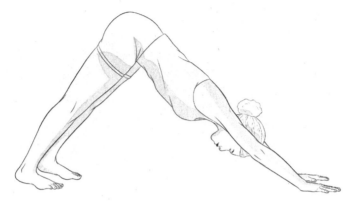

Overview: This pose mimics our furry friends by sending the tail up toward the sky and bowing the head down toward the ground, creating a profound overall stretch for the body. Just as in Cow pose and Cat pose, our hands become our feet in Downward-Facing Dog. This posture changes our perspective on the world around us and powerfully shifts the consciousness within us.

How-to: From Cat pose, walk your hands 1–2 inches in front of your shoulders. Curl your toes into the mat. Firmly press your hands into the floor, lift your hips up, and back away from the floor. Begin to straighten your legs as best you can without losing the length of your spine. Align your heels behind the widest part of your feet and release your heels toward the floor. Straighten your elbows, relax your head and your neck, and breathe fully in and out.

Benefits: Physically, this pose stretches the hamstrings, the calves, the feet, the shoulder girdle, and the wrists. It helps to relieve tension in the neck, and strengthens the quadriceps and the upper body. It is also a mild inversion, so it brings blood flow to the brain.

Energetically, Downward-Facing Dog opens the back gates of all chakras but specifically targets the first, fifth, and sixth of these energy centers. It helps us stay grounded while also enabling us to see things from a new perspective. This pose helps to release the unconscious energy lodged in the backs of the legs. It can help calm the mind, relieve stress, and reduce anxiety.

Engage *uddiyana* and *jalandhara bandha* to facilitate the movement of energy up to the crown. Engage *ashvini mudra* to create length in the spine. Increases *udana vayu*.

Therapeutic applications: This pose helps with carpal tunnel syndrome and relieves headaches, insomnia, back pain, and fatigue. It can help reduce high blood pressure and asthma, relieves flat feet, and is helpful for sciatica and sinusitis. Downward-Facing Dog can also be therapeutic for compressed or bulging discs by creating traction in the spine and neck.

Helpful tips: If your hamstrings are tight, take the feet wider than hip-distance apart and/or bend both knees so the spine can lengthen. If your shoulders are tight, take your hands slightly wider than shoulder-distance apart and point the fingertips out toward the corner edges of your mat. If you have wrist or shoulder injuries, or are fatigued in Downward-Facing Dog, try Child's Pose, *Balasana,* as an alternative: Lower the knees to the floor and move your seat back toward your heels. Rest your belly onto your thighs, your elbows onto the floor, and your forehead onto the mat. Rest here, allowing the weight of your body to release to the floor.

PLANK POSE:
PHALAKASANA

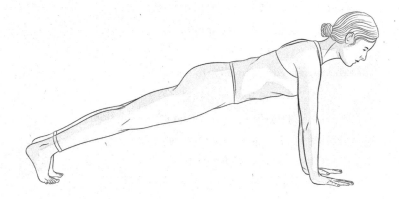

Overview: This posture teaches us how to build resilience through a strong core while harnessing the free flow of the breath. We are reminded of how capable we are of moving through challenges and that clarity often comes when we stay present with them.

How-to: From Downward-Facing Dog pose, shift your weight forward so that your shoulders line up over your wrists and your hips line up with your shoulders. Lift the tops of your thighs and keep your gaze fixed on the front edge of your mat. Stretch your heels toward the wall behind you as you reach the center of your chest forward, toward the wall in front of you. Lift your navel toward the spine and broaden across the collarbones. Breathe fully in and out.

Benefits: Physically, this posture strengthens the quadriceps, the pelvic floor, the lower abdominal muscles, the obliques, the forearms, and the upper body. It stretches the wrists.

Energetically, Plank pose builds *tapas*. It works on the third chakra, generating a sense of will, courage, and self-empowerment. It also helps tone the pelvic floor to strengthen *mula bandha*.

Engage *mula* and *uddiyana bandha*. Increases *samana vayu*.

Therapeutic applications: Plank pose can help reduce lower back pain by strengthening the core. It helps boost metabolism and can aid in reducing obesity.

Helpful tips: If you cannot sustain this pose without sinking in the lower back or straining your breath, lower the knees to the floor. If you have a wrist injury, lower your forearms to the floor. Place a block in between the thighs to awaken the muscles of the legs.

LOW PUSH-UP POSE:
CHATURANGA DANDASANA

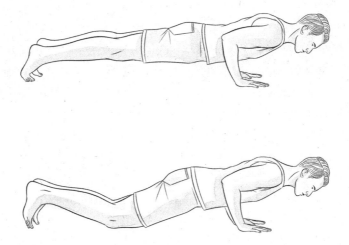

Overview: This pose is often practiced in transition, sandwiched between Plank and Upward-Facing Dog pose, commonly known as a *vinyasa.* Rarely performed on its own, Low Push-Up pose tends to be practiced quickly, without attention to alignment, which leads to injury. When done correctly, this pose not only strengthens the core and the upper body but also teaches us about collaboration. By recruiting multiple muscle groups to work together in harmony, we learn how to be efficient with our energy and intentional with our body.

How-to: From Plank pose, shift your weight a little forward toward the tips of your toes without dropping the hips. Keep your

gaze forward, toward the front edge of your mat, and bend your elbows straight back, keeping the tops of the shoulders lifting away
from the floor. Lower your whole body toward the mat until your
shoulders meet your elbows. Keep lifting your inner thighs and draw
your navel toward the spine. Move the shoulder blades in toward one
another and away from the ears. Stay in this position and breathe.

Benefits: Physically, Low Push-Up pose strengthens the legs, the
core, the arms, and the upper body.

Energetically, this pose develops tenacity, discipline, and inner
strength. It stimulates the third chakra, stoking the inner fire of will
and transformation.

Engage *mula* and slight *uddiyana bandha.* Stimulates *samana vayu.*

Therapeutic applications: Great for strength building and stabilizing the shoulder girdle; helps reduce lethargy and mild depression.

Helpful tips: If your hips and core sink below your shoulders, lower
the knees to the floor to support the lower belly. Place a block underneath your lower abdomen for support and to align the shoulder girdle. Place a block in between the thighs to activate the legs.

BACKBENDS

Our bodies are conditioned to lean forward toward what we see. Many of us spend a good portion of our days crouching over our desks, looking down at our phones, or reaching for the steering wheel of our cars. Back-bending is a powerful way to counter poor posture and move us into the space we cannot see. Backbends open the path of *rajas*, which is energizing, uplifting, and motivating. They expose us to the outside world, which can make us feel both vulnerable and liberated at the same time. Backbends can also help us connect to the emotions that surface in the heart: openness, compassion, sensitivity, and unconditional love.

BABY COBRA POSE:
BHUJANGASANA

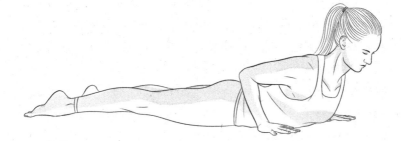

Overview: Although many versions of Cobra pose exist, this one is the safest and most therapeutic for the lower back. It builds strength and flexibility so that, like a snake, we develop mobility, stealth, and grace.

How-to: From a prone position, facing the floor, place your hands on either side of your chest and spread your fingers wide. Stretch your toes toward the wall behind you and press all ten toenails into the floor. As you inhale, lift your chest, neck, and head up off the floor. Lift your inner thighs toward the ceiling and relax the buttocks. Keep your shoulder blades moving away from your ears and lengthen the back of your neck. Breathe smoothly in and out.

Benefits: Physically, Baby Cobra pose strengthens the hamstrings, the buttocks, and the muscles along the spine. It stretches the abdomen, the lungs, the chest, and the shoulders. *Bhujangasana* also stimulates the digestive organs.

Energetically, this pose is uplifting and stimulating. It activates the fourth chakra, building on our capacity to experience compassion, connection, and unconditional love. This pose also frees the breath and helps activate the inhalation.

Engage slight *mula bandha* and *jalandhara bandha* to keep alignment in the neck. Engage *vajroli mudra* to encourage length in the spine. Increases *prana vayu*.

Therapeutic applications: Can help with mild depression, asthma, poor posture, and scoliosis.

Helpful tips: Place a block between the ankles or the inner thighs to help align the legs. Avoid this pose if you have any wrist sensitivity.

UPWARD-FACING DOG POSE:
URDVA MUKHA SVANASANA

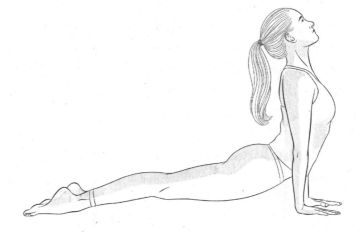

Overview: Although this posture is often practiced as part of the Sun Salutation series, there are many benefits to practicing it independently. By opening the space at the center of the chest and lifting our gaze toward the sky, this pose creates freedom as the heart awakens us to infinite intelligence.

How-to: From Baby Cobra pose, slide the hands down a couple of inches toward the waist. Press the hands firmly into the floor and straighten the elbows, lifting the knees, the thighs, the hips, and the belly off the floor. Roll the shoulder blades back and down, away from the ears. Lift through the inner thighs and draw the lower abdomen toward the spine. Look toward the ceiling, keeping the back of your neck long.

Benefits: Physically, Upward-Facing Dog pose stretches the quadriceps, the hip flexors, the abdomen, the chest, the shoulders, and the throat. It strengthens the upper body and stimulates the digestive organs.

Energetically, this pose encourages inhalation and our capacity to take a full breath. It strongly activates the fourth chakra, promoting a quality of external connection, emotional sensitivity, compassion, and love.

Engage *mula bandha* and *vajroli mudra*. Increases *prana vayu*.

Therapeutic applications: Can alleviate mild depression, kyphosis (forward rounding of the back), and sluggish digestion.

Helpful tips: Stay with Baby Cobra pose if you have any wrist or lower back issues. Place a block between the thighs to help create more space in the lower back.

FLYING LOCUST POSE:
SALABHASANA

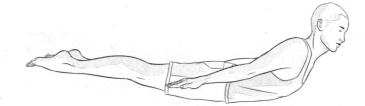

Overview: Often referred to as "superhero pose" by children, Flying Locust pose taps into the superpower of our resistance to gravity. While it creates freedom in the chest and shoulders, this posture is a humble reminder of the power of that downward force and the strength it takes for our whole back body to move against it.

How-to: From a prone position, facing the floor, extend your arms down alongside your body with the palms facing down. Bring your forehead to the floor and press the tops of your feet down. On your inhalation, lift your chest, neck, and head off the floor. Then stretch back through your toes and lift the legs from the inner thighs. Now raise your hands off the floor. Lengthen your tailbone back toward your heels. Reach the center of the chest toward the wall in front of you. Align the shoulder blades on your back, keep the back of your neck long. Stay in this position and breathe in and out.

Benefits: Physically, Flying Locust pose strengthens the hamstrings, the buttocks, and the back. It opens the shoulders, the chest, and the thighs. It helps correct poor posture and stimulates digestion.

Additionally, strengthening the back body helps to create space for the organs to function correctly.

Energetically, this pose opens the fourth chakra, which governs our emotions and enables us to feel compassion for others. It also helps build our sense of autonomy by strengthening the muscles along the spine, which helps us to stand tall and erect. Lastly, this pose facilitates a long spine, which, energetically, enables us to feel the central channel of the spine, or *brahma nadi.*

Engage *mula bandha* and *vajroli mudra.* Engage slight *jalandhara bandha* to keep length in the back of the neck. Stimulates *prana vayu.*

Therapeutic applications: Alleviates fatigue, indigestion, lower back pain, scoliosis.

Helpful tips: Place a block in between the thighs to help create more space in the lower back. To open the shoulders, practice this pose while clasping the fingers behind you at the small of the back.

BOW POSE:
DHANURASANA

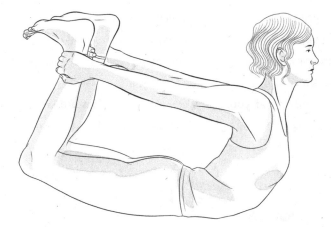

Overview: Like the bow that helps an arrow take flight, this pose helps liberate the individual spirit at the center of the chest, known as the *jiva atman*. When the *jiva* is liberated, we can feel a sense of connection to all beings.

How-to: From Flying Locust pose, bend both legs and take hold of the ankles or the toes. Press back through your shins and begin to lift the inner thighs, the torso, and the chest off the floor. Lengthen your tailbone back toward your heels and keep the back of your neck long. Breathe in and out into the chest.

Benefits: Physically, this pose stretches the quadriceps, the hip flexors, the abdomen, the chest, the shoulders, and the biceps. It strengthens the gluteal muscles and the hamstrings, and stimulates the digestive organs.

Energetically, Bow pose opens the fourth chakra. Because it so significantly opens the front of the body, it increases the quality of *rajas*, which is the energy that awakens us and projects us into the future.

Engage *mula bandha* and *vajroli mudra*. Stimulates *prana vayu*.

Therapeutic applications: Stimulates digestion, can help boost metabolism, combats depression, helps alleviate upper respiratory congestion and asthma.

Helpful tips: If your quadriceps or hip flexors are tight, try this pose with your torso close to the floor. If you have any shoulder sensitivity, keep your arms alongside your body or practice holding on to your feet with a strap.

BRIDGE POSE:
SETU BANDHA SARVANGASANA

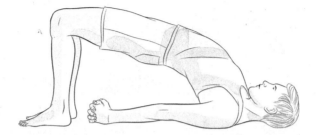

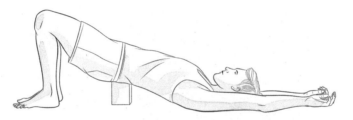

Overview: Like a daily vitamin, this pose helps boost our immune system and regulate our energy levels when done regularly. It stretches muscles that are tight and strengthens weak muscles, creating a harmonious effect on our body, mind, and nervous system.

How-to: From Constructive Rest pose (see page 276), place your arms alongside your body and your feet into a parallel position. Walk your heels in so that they almost touch your fingertips. Inhale and lift your hips off the floor, pressing down into the big toe mound of the foot. Interlace your fingers underneath you, work the shoulder blades toward one another, and bring your palms together to touch. Lift your chin away from your chest as you lift your chest toward your chin.

Benefits: Physically, this pose is very similar to Flying Locust pose in that it strengthens the hamstrings, the buttocks, and the back, and it also supports the quadriceps. It opens the shoulders, the chest, the thighs, and the hip flexors, and helps correct poor posture. This pose also stimulates the abdominal organs, the lungs, and the thyroid gland.

Energetically, this pose opens the fourth chakra. It is energizing, frees the breath, and can help cure mild depression.

Engage *mula* and *jalandhara bandha* and *vajroli mudra*. Stimulates *prana vayu*.

Therapeutic applications: This pose can be helpful in alleviating asthma, high blood pressure, osteoporosis, and sinusitis, and is helpful with postnatal conditions. It regulates the thymus and the thyroid gland. When done with a block under the sacrum, this pose can help ease menstrual disorders.

Helpful tips: Place a block in between the thighs to help create space in the lower back. If your shoulders are tight, keep your arms alongside your body or hold on to the outer edges of your mat. For a more restorative option, place a block or a thick cushion underneath your sacrum.

CAMEL POSE:
USTRASANA

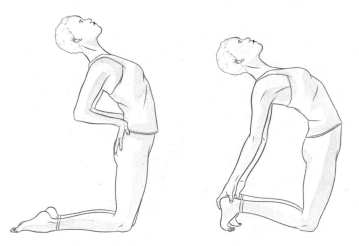

Overview: As one of the more intense chest openers, Camel pose gives a natural boost to your mood and energy level. Not only does it free up space in the chest, but it frees the breath and the *jiva*—the individual spirit—as well, creating a feeling of expansiveness and liberation.

How-to: From a kneeling position, align your hips directly over your knees and your shoulders over your hips. Place the hands on the lower back, fingertips pointing either toward the chest or down toward the floor. Engage your lower abdomen and lift your chest away from your navel as if you had a thread pulling your sternum up toward the ceiling. Curl your toes into the floor. Reach for your heels with your fingertips, keeping your hips stacked over the knees. Keep the back of your neck long and breathe.

Benefits: Physically, Camel pose stretches the quadriceps, the hip flexors, the chest, the shoulders, and the throat. It strengthens the backs of the legs and the muscles along the spine, while stimulating the adrenals, the kidneys, and the digestive organs. This pose also helps to correct poor posture.

Energetically, *Ustrasana* is mood-boosting and bolsters stamina. It stimulates the fourth and fifth chakras, enhancing our confidence and our ability to connect to the outside world, communicating our truth with love and compassion.

Engage *mula* and slight *jalandhara bandha* to keep the back of the neck long. Engage *vajroli mudra*. Stimulates *prana vayu*.

Therapeutic applications: Helps with kyphosis, asthma, mild depression, neck pain, and lower back pain. Indicated for women during pregnancy.

Helpful tips: Place a blanket under the knees if your kneecaps are sensitive. Put a block in between the thighs to help engage *mula bandha*. Place a large bolster or blocks on your calves to bridge the gap between the feet and the hands and to keep the backbend in the thoracic spine.

INVERSIONS

Two of the most common inversions in yoga—Headstand and Shoulder Stand—were traditionally referred to as the king and queen of all the poses because they encourage the union of Shakti, the divine feminine force at the base of the spine, to Shiva, pure consciousness at the crown. When these two forces converge, yoga happens. Inversions take us into the unknown, moving us out of our comfort zone and into our fears, which helps us see both the world and ourselves from a new perspective.

DOLPHIN POSE:
SALAMBA SIRSASANA

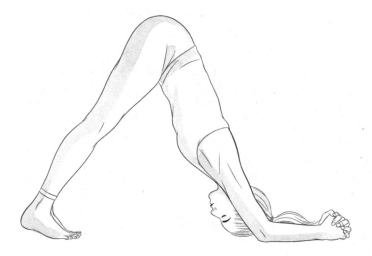

Overview: Like Downward-Facing Dog pose, this pose is a mild inversion. It is a helpful preparation for Headstand, with many of the same benefits and not as many of the risk factors. If you feel stuck in your ways, try this posture to shift how you perceive the world.

How-to: From hands and knees, lower each forearm down onto the floor to align the elbows directly underneath the shoulders. Interlace your fingers and press your forearms and outer wrists into the floor as you curl your toes into the mat. Lift your hips up, away from the floor, and walk your feet in slightly closer, toward the face. Stay and breathe, letting your head and neck relax toward the floor.

Benefits: Physically, this pose opens the calves, the hamstrings, and the shoulders. It strengthens the upper body and the back, and helps bring blood to the brain, increasing mental alertness.

Energetically, Dolphin pose helps us to see things from a new perspective. It stimulates the fourth, fifth, and sixth chakras, facilitating a release at the heart, clear communication, and mental focus.

Energetic tip: When coming out of the pose, pause and sit back on your heels, feeling the reversal of the upward and downward passages. Like two rivers converging, these passages meet at the center of the chest, liberating the *jiva atman,* the individual spirit that connects us with all things.

Engage *mula bandha, uddiyana bandha,* and *ashvini mudra.* Stimulates *udana vayu.*

Therapeutic applications: Relieves mild headaches, fatigue, sinusitis, and mild depression.

Helpful tips: If you have any shoulder sensitivity or high or low blood pressure, practice *Viparita Karani* (see page 278).

HEADSTAND:
SIRSASANA

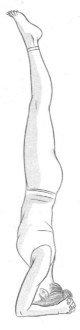

Overview: Traditionally known as the "king of all poses," Headstand opens the crown chakra, which is the energy center that connects us to infinite intelligence. Although many risk factors come with practicing Headstand, it can powerfully shift our mind, body, and consciousness when done safely. By reversing our relationship to the Earth, *Sirsasana* also reverses the flow of gravity in our body and changes how we relate to the world and to ourselves.

How-to: From Dolphin pose, lower the knees onto the floor. Switch the position of your head, so that the crown of your head touches the floor. Interlace the fingers behind your head and press your forearms into the floor, lifting your shoulders up, away from the ears. Walk your feet in as close to your face as you can. Bend one knee and then the other toward the chest. Lift your tailbone and slowly begin to extend your legs toward the ceiling, pressing through the balls of the feet, and peeling the toes back. Stay and breathe for as long as you can without strain. Please note that you should not practice this pose for the first time without the guidance of a teacher or an expert, especially if you have any preexisting neck, shoulder, or blood pressure conditions.

Benefits: Physically, Headstand strengthens the legs, the pelvic floor, the abdomen, and the back, and opens the chest and the shoulders. This pose stimulates the pituitary and pineal glands in the brain and improves digestion, while helping to improve lymphatic circulation and venous blood flow to the heart. It can also reduce swelling in the feet and ankles.

Energetically, *Sirsasana* moves us into our fears and helps to shift our perspective. It stimulates the sixth and seventh chakras, harnessing the qualities of insight and innovation while also promoting our connection to unbound intelligence. Engage *mula, uddiyana,* and *jalandhara bandha.* Stimulates *udana vayu.*

Therapeutic applications: Relieves headaches, sinusitis, asthma, insomnia, infertility, edema, and mild depression; helpful for postnatal conditions.

Helpful tips: Practice at the wall to help with balance. If you have any neck injuries, practice Dolphin pose or, alternatively, place two or three blocks underneath each shoulder and bend at your elbows so that the elbows align underneath each shoulder. Place your hands in front of the blocks and spread the fingers wide. Kick one foot up at a time so the legs are either against a wall or up toward the ceiling.

SHOULDER STAND:
SARVANGASANA

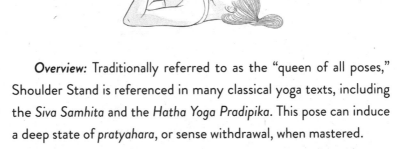

Overview: Traditionally referred to as the "queen of all poses," Shoulder Stand is referenced in many classical yoga texts, including the *Siva Samhita* and the *Hatha Yoga Pradipika*. This pose can induce a deep state of *pratyahara*, or sense withdrawal, when mastered.

How-to: Lying flat on your back, extend your arms alongside your body with the palms facing down. Inhale, and on your exhale, use your abdominal muscles to lift your legs so that your feet touch the floor behind you. Curl the toes under and lift your hips away from your shoulders. Draw your shoulder blades toward one another and bend your elbows, placing your palms flat on your upper back. Lift one leg toward the ceiling followed by the other one, pressing through the balls of the feet and peeling the toes back. Stay here and breathe.

Benefits: Physically, Shoulder Stand strengthens the legs and the core. It stretches and supports the back, stretches the shoulders and the back of the neck, helps regulate the thyroid gland, and aids in digestion. Shoulder Stand also helps improve lymphatic circulation and venous blood flow to the heart. It can also help reduce swelling in the feet and ankles.

Energetically, this pose reduces anxiety and calms the nervous system by stimulating the parasympathetic nerves at the back of the neck. It helps induce *pratyahara*, or sense withdrawal, bringing us into a deep state of quiet and introspection. Shoulder Stand stimulates the fifth and sixth chakras, facilitating our ability to be silent, communicate with clarity, and build insight, intuition, and higher vision.

Engage *mula, uddiyana,* and *jalandhara bandha.* Increases *udana vayu.*

Therapeutic applications: Shoulder Stand reduces anxiety, high blood pressure, and varicose veins. It alleviates thyroid imbalances, insomnia, and edema, and can ease the symptoms of menopause.

Helpful tips: Place a flat, folded blanket underneath your shoulders to create more space in the back of your neck. If you have any neck sensitivity, avoid this pose and practice Legs Up the Wall pose instead (see page 278).

PLOW POSE:
HALASANA

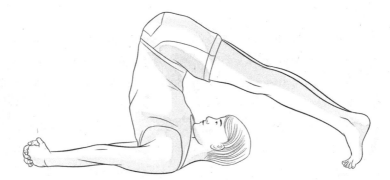

Overview: As a physical shape, Plow pose is like Staff pose (see page 266), rotated 180 degrees. It evokes the same qualities as a Seated Forward Bend with the added benefit of inverting. This pose can elicit profound physical, mental, and energetic responses that lead to a deep state of awareness when done safely.

How-to: From Shoulder Stand, bend at your hips and allow your feet to lower down toward the floor overhead. Keep your toes curled into the floor. Lift your tailbone toward the ceiling and release your hands and elbows toward the floor. Draw your shoulder blades in toward one another and interlace your fingers, bringing your palms to touch so that your upper and lower arms are firmly pressing into the floor. Lift your chest toward your chin and your chin away from your chest. Stay here and breathe.

Benefits: Physically, Plow pose stretches the hamstrings, the lower back, the upper back, and the back of the neck. It also extends the chest, the shoulders, and the upper arms. This pose strengthens the abdomen and the muscles along the spine. It also regulates the thyroid gland.

Energetically, this pose is calming and cooling. It activates the first and fifth chakras, creating a deep release in the unconscious through the hamstrings while also cultivating an internal space of silence for clear, unbridled communication at the throat.

Engage *mula, uddiyana,* and *jalandhara bandha.* Increases *udana vayu.*

Therapeutic applications: This pose relieves lower backache, headache, fatigue, insomnia, and sinusitis. It helps to ease symptoms of menopause and to maintain thyroid regulation.

Helpful tips: If you feel tension in the back of your neck, place a carefully folded blanket underneath the upper back to create more space in the cervical spine. Place a strap or a belt around the upper arms to keep the elbows from splaying away from one another. Place a bolster or a chair underneath your toes if your hamstrings are tight. If you have any cervical spine injuries, practice *Paschimottanasana* (see page 272) instead.

SEATED TWISTS

Not only do seated twists aid in our digestion and in keeping the spine healthy, but they also help to flush old blood out of our organs and bring in fresh blood. This squeeze-and-soak action is cleansing and detoxifying, and it allows us to let go of what is no longer serving us so that we can awaken to new possibilities.

HALF LORD OF THE FISHES POSE:
ARDHA MATSYENDRASANA

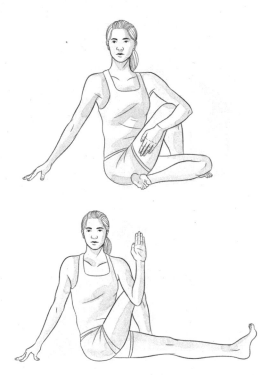

Overview: According to the *Hatha Yoga Pradipika* (1.26–27), this pose is meant to destroy many diseases. Although modern science might dispute that, this pose keeps the spine strong, aligned, and lengthened. The ancient yogis considered the integrity of the spine a measure of proper health, as it supports the flow of breath and life force energy.

How-to: From Staff pose (see page 266), bend the right leg, and cross the right foot over the left leg, so that the sole of the right foot is on the floor to the outside of the left sit bone. Roll the left thigh open toward the left and place the left foot to the outside of the right sit bone. Root down evenly through both sit bones. Hug the right knee with the left arm. As you inhale, reach the right arm toward the ceiling. On the exhale, lower the arm down behind you, resting the fingertips on the floor behind you. Lengthen your spine as you inhale, and rotate around the axis of your spine as you exhale, keeping your chest lifted and the shoulder blades moving in toward one another and down the back. Allow the crown of the head to lengthen toward the ceiling as you root down evenly into both sit bones.

Benefits: Physically, this pose strengthens the obliques, the abdominal muscles, and the back. It stretches the external rotators of the hips and the shoulder girdle. The pose aids in digestion by massaging the internal organs and, like a sponge, gently compresses and plumps up the intervertebral discs, leading to a longer, healthier spine.

Energetically, this pose stimulates the third chakra, which strengthens and promotes transformation. It stimulates the *agni*, the digestive fire of conversion that helps us metabolize our food and process our thoughts and feelings. This pose can also help release stagnant energy by rinsing out blood from the organs and bringing in fresh blood and renewed energy.

Engage *mula, uddiyana,* and *jalandhara bandha.* Stimulates *samana vayu.*

Therapeutic applications: Alleviates constipation, sluggish digestion, asthma, sciatica, scoliosis, and lower backache.

Helpful tip: If your hips are tight and your spine is rounded, either sit on a blanket or keep the lower leg extended straight out to get more length in the spine.

RECLINED TWIST POSE:
JATHARA PARIVARTANASANA

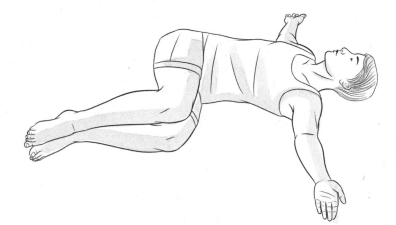

Overview: This calming and therapeutic pose is excellent for regulating the nervous system, relieving lower back pain, and learning the art of surrender. Once you come into the shape of the pose, let the pose do the work for you.

How-to: From Constructive Rest pose (see page 276), walk the feet in so that they come directly underneath your knees. Take your arms wide in a "T" shape and align your wrists with your shoulders. Inhale and lift your hips, shift them over to the right a couple of inches, and lower them back down. Lift your feet off the floor and drop them over to the left so that you make a right angle with your hips, knees, and ankles. Take hold of the top right thigh with your left hand to keep the legs stacked and either keep your gaze toward the ceiling or over your right arm.

Benefits: Physically, this pose stretches the outer hips, the illiotibial (IT) band, the hamstrings, the lower back, the chest, and the shoulders. It aids in the digestive process by massaging the digestive organs.

Energetically, Reclined Twist pose works on the third chakra to help stoke the digestive fire. A relatively passive pose, it connects us to our more lunar, feminine energy.

Engage slight *jalandhara bandha.* Stimulates *samana vayu.*

Therapeutic applications: Relieves scoliosis, lower back pain, fatigue, and constipation, and eases the pain of osteoporosis.

Helpful tips: Place a blanket in between the knees if your hips are tight. Place a blanket underneath the extended arm if your shoulders are tight. For a deeper stretch in the hamstrings and outer hips, keep the legs straight.

SEATED HIP OPENERS

This category of poses stimulates the second chakra, which is governed by the element of water. Water gives rise to taste, feeling, creativity, sensuality, and sexuality. Because the hips are the energetic storehouse of our unprocessed emotions, deep hip openers can release suppressed feelings when we hold them for an extended period of time. By freeing up this region of the body, we allow ourselves to experience our feelings more fully, which helps us to show up more wholly.

RECLINED PIGEON POSE:
SUPTA KAPOTASANA

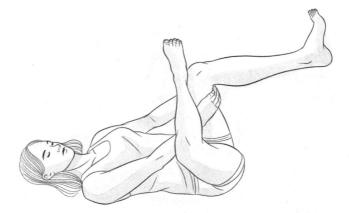

Overview: This profound stretch releases our hips and lower back, leading to greater overall ease and mobility. By locating our aware-ness on one single point of sensation, we enter the stage of *dharana*, relaxed concentration.

How-to: From Constructive Rest pose (see page 276), cross your right ankle on top of your left thigh. Flex the right foot to engage the muscles around the knee joint. Interlace your fingers behind the left thigh and lift the left foot off the floor, gently drawing your left thigh closer toward you as you consciously move your right thigh away from your body. Stay here and breathe, resting your awareness in the area where you feel sensation in the body.

Benefits: Physically, *Supta Kapotasana* stretches the hamstrings, the outer hips, and the piriformis muscle.

Energetically, this pose calms the nervous system and relaxes the mind. It stimulates the second chakra, freeing up unprocessed emotions, which prompts creativity, sensuality, and sexuality.

Engage slight *jalandhara bandha*. Stimulates *apana* and *vyana vayu*.

Therapeutic applications: Relieves lower back pain and sciatica; suitable for pregnant practitioners in their first and second trimesters.

Helpful tips: If you cannot reach the back of the leg with the hands, use a strap, or lower the foot to the floor or rest it against a chair.

BOUND ANGULAR POSE:
BADDHA KONASANA

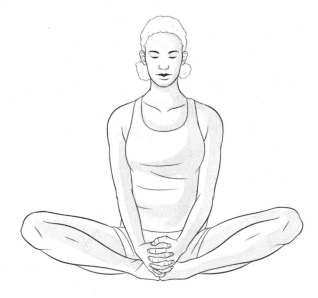

Overview: This pose, often referred to as "Cobbler's pose," is commonly assumed by the shoemakers and other artisans of India. Because the Western population is used to sitting in chairs, finding comfort in Bound Angular pose may be challenging. In addition to providing a deep stretch in the hips, it teaches us how to find grace in awkward and uncomfortable situations.

How-to: From Staff pose (see page 266), bring the soles of your feet together and spread your knees wide apart. Adjust the flesh of your buttocks so that you are sitting on your sit bones and not on your tailbone. Inhale and lengthen your spine. As you exhale, begin to hinge forward at your hips, keeping your spine long and your shoulders away from your ears. Continue to breathe your way into the pose: Inhale, lengthen; exhale, deepen.

Benefits: Physically, this pose stretches the knees, the inner thighs, the outer hips, the lower back.

Through the lengthening of the inhale and the deepening of the exhale, we learn how to be guided by the breath and not the ego. Energetically, Bound Angular pose teaches the qualities of deep reflection and contemplation. This pose stimulates the second chakra, cultivating the qualities of fluidity, flexibility, sexuality, and sensuality.

Engage *mula bandha, uddiyana bandha,* and *jalandhara bandha.* Engage *ashvini mudra.* Stimulates *apana* and *vyana vayu.*

Therapeutic applications: This pose soothes menstrual discomfort and sciatica. It relieves lower back pain and symptoms of menopause, stimulates the reproductive organs, and increases sexual energy.

Helpful tips: If your hips or lower back are tight, place a blanket underneath your sit bones. If you have any knee sensitivity, place a block underneath each knee.

EASY SEAT:
SUKHASANA

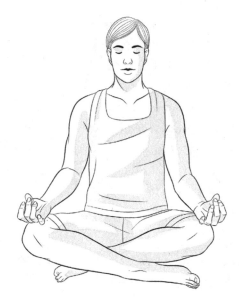

Overview: Easy Seat is most often used for meditation and contemplation. The Sanskrit word *sukha* is translated as "sweetness" or "ease." Although this pose may not be inherently easy for all bodies, it is in our approach to the posture that the most significant benefits are reaped. Easy Seat reminds us that the path to joy is joy itself.

How-to: From Staff pose (see page 266), rotate your right thigh open and place your right foot in toward your groin. Rotate your left thigh open and put your left foot in front of the right foot, sitting in a cross-legged position. Adjust the flesh of your buttocks so that you are sitting on your sit bones and not your tailbone. Now allow the torso to naturally lengthen away from the pelvis, using the abdominal muscles to support the lower back and the muscles along the spine to support the upper back. Relax the tops of the shoulders and feel the head and neck naturally floating atop the spine. Rest your hands on your knees and relax your facial muscles.

Benefits: Physically, Easy Seat stretches the hips and the knees, strengthens the muscles along the spine, tones the abdominal muscles, and supports good posture.

Energetically, Easy Seat helps us to feel grounded, steady, and at ease, all at the same time. This is an excellent pose to assume for breathwork and other contemplative practices. It opens the second and sixth chakras and the central channel that connects the lower and upper consciousness, known as *sushumna nadi.*

Engage *mula bandha.* Stimulates *apana* and *vyana vayu.*

Therapeutic applications: Alleviates lower back pain, helps with perimenopause and menopause, reduces tension in the mind.

Helpful tips: If your hips or lower back are tight, place a blanket or a cushion underneath your sit bones. If your knees are sensitive, place a block underneath each knee.

ONE-LEGGED PIGEON POSE:
EKA PADA KAPOTASANA

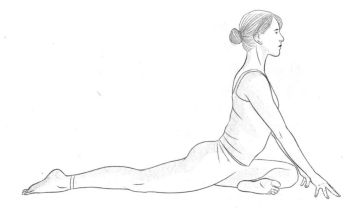

Overview: One-Legged Pigeon pose deeply releases the layers of tension that accumulate in the physical and subtle body. It targets the outer hips and the psoas muscle, both of which carry the responsibilities of stabilizing and connecting the upper and lower body. When we allow ourselves to surrender into this pose, we create a sense of unburdening from within, freeing ourselves to feel, breathe, and be.

How-to: From Downward-Facing Dog pose, inhale and lift your right leg up and back behind you. As you exhale, bend your right knee toward your chest. Flex your right foot and lower your ankle, shin, and knee down in between your hands. Keep the back toes curled under and press your hands into the floor to lift your hips off the mat, drawing your right hip back and your left hip forward. Uncurl the back toes and inhale as you engage your lower belly, lifting your chest and your gaze toward the ceiling. As you exhale, lower your torso down toward the floor, lowering your head either to the mat or onto a block.

Benefits: Physically, One-Legged Pigeon pose stretches the ankles, the quadriceps, the psoas, the inner thighs, the outer hips, and the back.

Energetically, this pose helps to reduce tension in the mind. It works on the second chakra, freeing both emotional and sexual energy to help increase creativity and our sensory connection to the world. It also helps free the breath by stretching the psoas muscle.

Engage slight *jalandhara bandha.* Stimulates *apana* and *vyana vayu.*

Therapeutic applications: Alleviates lower back pain, addresses urinary disorders, improves posture, helps ease the symptoms of perimenopause and menopause, and eases sciatica.

Helpful tips: Place a cushion or a pillow underneath your torso for a more therapeutic variation. If you have any ankle, knee, or hip sensitivity, practice Reclined Pigeon pose instead. If your hips are off the floor, place a rolled towel or a cushion underneath your lifted sit bone.

FIRE LOG POSE:
AGNISTAMBHASANA

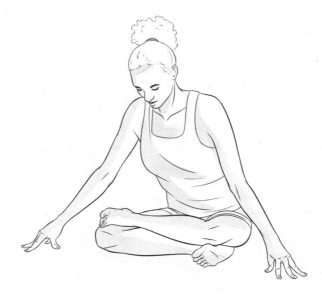

Overview: Fire Log pose targets the deep external rotators in the hips, which help to stabilize us. Because this shape yields such an intense physical response in the body, it teaches us how to rest in the awareness of what we are feeling without judgment or manipulation. As we become more aware of our sensations, the sensations shift and dissolve into awareness itself.

How-to: From Bound Angular pose, take hold of the right foot with both hands and gently place the right ankle on top of the left thigh. Stack the right shin on top of the left shin so that the ankles and knees are aligned directly on top of each other. Anchor your sit bones down into the floor as you lengthen your spine toward the ceiling. Stay here or begin to fold forward over the legs, deepening the stretch in the outer hips.

Benefits: Physically, Fire Log pose stretches the knees, the inner thighs, the outer hips, and the lower back.

Energetically, this pose helps to reduce tension in the mind. It works on the second chakra, freeing both emotional and sexual energy to help increase creativity and our sensory connection to the world.

Engage *mula bandha.* Stimulates *apana* and *vyana vayu.*

Therapeutic applications: Alleviates lower back pain, helps relieve the symptoms of perimenopause and menopause, and eases sciatica.

Helpful tips: If your hips or lower back are tight, place a blanket or a cushion underneath your sit bones. If your knees are sensitive, place a block underneath the top knee or practice *Supta Kapotasana* (see page 254) instead.

SEATED FORWARD BENDS

Although a growing number of humans sit for most of the day, we do not necessarily know how to sit in a way that's healthy for our spine and our organs. This category of poses teaches us how to keep the spine aligned, the breath balanced, and the organs spacious in a seated position. Energetically, seated forward bends open the back of the body, which activates the passage of *tamas*, the quieting, pacifying part of our body. They also deeply stretch the hamstrings, which energetically store a lot of our patterning and limiting beliefs. For this reason, seated forward bends are a profound way to close the physical practice. They actively help free us from bondage, transitioning our minds from the outer, sensory world to an internal, quiet space of pure consciousness.

STAFF POSE:
DANDASANA

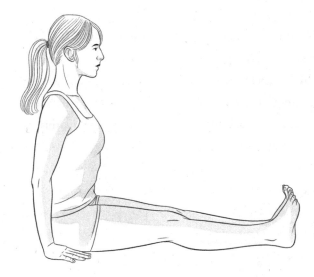

Overview: Staff pose is to the seated poses what Mountain pose is to the standing poses. In the case of Staff pose, the sit bones are like our feet, anchoring and rooting us to the Earth, while the spine rises toward the sky. Practicing Staff pose every day not only strengthens the core and stabilizes the spine but also empowers us to hold ourselves up from the center of our being, establishing a sense of autonomy, individuation, and connection to pure potential.

How-to: From a seated position, extend both legs out in front of you. Adjust your seat from side to side, so you feel your sit bones and not your tailbone on the floor. Engage your quadriceps and spread your toes. Lengthen your spine toward the ceiling, stacking your rib cage over your pelvis and your shoulders over your rib cage. Keep your hands alongside your body and create space across your collar-bones, softening the tops of the shoulders and releasing them away from your ears. Allow your head and neck to float freely atop your spine.

Benefits: Physically, Staff pose strengthens the legs, the core, and the upper back. It stretches the calves, the hamstrings, the chest, and the shoulders.

Energetically, this pose is both grounding and liberating. By balancing the front and the back of the body evenly, this pose takes us into *satva guna*. It activates the first and third chakras, creating steadiness, stability, and self-empowerment from within. Staff pose helps position the spine, which also energetically aligns the two central channels that run along it: *sushumna* and *brahma nadis*. Stimulating these channels facilitates both manifestation and transcendence.

Engage *mula* and slight *uddiyana bandha*. Engage *ashvini mudra* to lengthen the front of the body. Stimulates *apana vayu*.

Therapeutic applications: Staff pose strengthens the core, which can be helpful for children with sensory processing issues. It also corrects poor posture, addresses osteoporosis and other bone deficiency issues, and relieves lower back conditions.

Helpful tips: If your hamstrings or lower back muscles are tight, place a blanket or a cushion underneath your seat. If your hamstrings are very restricted, bend the knees.

HEAD TO KNEE POSE:
JANUSIRSASANA

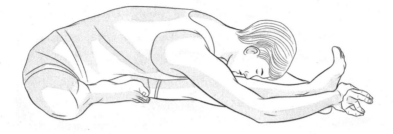

Overview: Although the English translation of this pose is "head to knee," we are actually lengthening our belly button to our knee and our head to our shin. This profoundly releasing pose opens the whole back of the body while also providing a slight twist over the extended leg. It is cleansing and replenishing, and it helps us to get unstuck as we move deeper inward to the essence of our being.

How-to: From Staff pose, bend the right leg, and externally rotate the right thigh open, placing the sole of the right foot on the inner left thigh. Inhale and lengthen the spine, rotating your torso over the extended left leg. As you exhale, hinge at your hips, keeping your lower belly engaged, your spine long, and your shoulders away from your ears. Continue to breathe your way into the pose, lengthening as you inhale and deepening over the extended leg as you exhale. Eventually, rest your abdomen onto your thigh, your forehead onto your shin, and your hands around the foot of the extended leg if that is available to you.

Benefits: Physically, Head to Knee pose stretches the hamstrings, the inner thighs, the outer hips, the lower back, the upper back, and the back of the neck. It helps with digestion and facilitates exhalation by gently compressing the diaphragm up.

Energetically, Head to Knee pose releases the unconscious patterning that gets locked in the backs of the legs. It stimulates the first chakra, creating a firm and solid connection to the Earth, facilitating a sense of freedom to release and let go with the exhalation. This pose helps us to detoxify ourselves, both physically and energetically, of what is no longer serving us. Opening the passage of *tamas* also calms and quiets the mind, encouraging a deep connection inward.

Engage *mula, uddiyana,* and *jalandhara bandha.* Engage *ashvini mudra* to lengthen the front of the body. Stimulates *apana vayu.*

Therapeutic applications: Head to Knee pose relieves scoliosis, lower back pain, menstrual discomfort, and symptoms of menopause. This pose can also alleviate headaches, anxiety, and fatigue, and improve digestion.

Helpful tips: If your hamstrings or lower back muscles are tight, place a blanket or a cushion underneath your seat. If your hands don't reach your foot, place a strap or a belt around the sole of the extended foot and continue to lengthen through the spine as you fold over the extended leg.

WIDE-ANGLE SEAT POSE:
UPAVISTA KONASANA

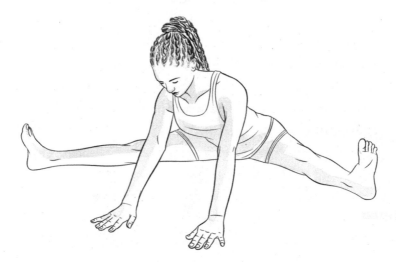

Overview: This pose can either be deeply releasing or deeply challenging, depending on your unique anatomy and constitution. Wide-Angle Seat pose can sometimes force us to confront our limitations, triggering frustration and discouragement. By surrendering our expectations and accepting our own personal range of motion, we can open to the grace of contentment and self-acceptance in this pose.

How-to: From Staff pose, open the legs wide in a "V" shape. Adjust the lower part of your thighs so you tilt at the pelvis and not at the waist. Place your hands either behind you or in front of you on the floor. As you inhale, lengthen your spine by firming your belly and lifting your chest. As you exhale, fold forward, lowering your torso toward the floor.

Benefits: Physically, Wide-Angle Seat pose stretches the calves, the hamstrings, the inner thighs, and the lower back. It strengthens the muscles along the spine and stimulates the abdominal organs.

Energetically, it activates the first and second chakras, creating strength and flexibility simultaneously. Opening the passage of *tamas* also calms and quiets the mind, encouraging a deep connection inward.

Engage *mula, uddiyana,* and *jalandhara bandha.* Engage *ashvini mudra* to lengthen the front of the body. Stimulates *apana vayu.*

Therapeutic applications: Relieves arthritis, sciatica, and lower back pain, and helps to detoxify the kidneys. It can relieve headaches, anxiety, and fatigue. Further, this pose helps address issues of menopause and menstrual discomfort, and prenatal discomfort.

Helpful tips: If your hamstrings or lower back muscles are tight, place a blanket or a cushion underneath your sit bones. Alternatively, bend the knees and place a small blanket roll or a block underneath each knee. If you have intense lower back pain, try this pose resting on your back with your sit bones up against the wall and your head away from the wall, taking your legs into a wide "V" shape.

STRETCH OF THE WEST POSE:
PASCHIMOTTANASANA

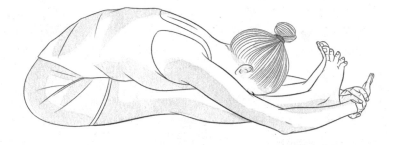

Overview: Like the peace and serenity that emerges from the setting sun, Stretch of the West pose cultivates a state of tranquility from within. Opening the back of the body and drawing our senses inward, we effortlessly transition from a state of doing to a state of being. This pose moves us from the more active, solar portion of the practice to the receptive, subtle-energetic space of contemplation.

How-to: From Staff pose, inhale and lengthen your spine. As you exhale, hinge at your hips, keeping your lower belly engaged, your spine long, and your shoulders away from your ears. Inhale and lengthen your spine, lifting your chest slightly and, as you exhale, release more deeply into the pose. Continue to breathe your way into the pose. If it is accessible to you, rest your belly on your thighs, your forehead on your shins, and your hands around the soles of the feet.

Benefits: Physically, Stretch of the West pose stretches the calves, the hamstrings, and the entire back of the body, including the

upper back and the back of the neck. It stimulates the liver, the kidneys, and the ovaries, and improves digestion.

Energetically, this pose moves us into *pratyahara*, the first stage
of Raja Yoga, which is the royal path that ultimately leads us to a state
of transcendence, or *samadhi*. Stretch of the West activates the first
and sixth chakras, deepening our connection to the Earth and facilitating a profound sense of surrender. By opening the passage of
tamas, this pose activates the back gates of all the chakras, drawing us
into the shadow side of our being. This enables us to face and integrate this shadow side into our consciousness and helps us achieve
insight and awareness.

Engage *mula*, *uddiyana*, and *jalandhara bandha*. Engage *ashvini
mudra* to lengthen the front of the body. Stimulates *apana vayu*.

Therapeutic applications: Stretch of the West pose relieves lower
back pain and helps detoxify the kidneys. This pose alleviates stress
and anxiety as well as symptoms of menopause and menstrual discomfort. It also offers relief for headaches and fatigue.

Helpful tips: If your hamstrings or lower back muscles are tight,
place a blanket or a cushion underneath your seat. Loop a strap or a
belt around the sole of the feet if you need a longer stretch.

RESTFUL/RESTORATIVE POSTURES

Our modern-day culture disproportionately emphasizes the heat-building, activating qualities of this practice, but there is another integral piece to the state of yoga: surrender. As a society, many of us are not taught how to relax. We are taught to be productive and goal-oriented, and to achieve goals at all costs. The authentic practice of yoga is an undoing of that belief system. It is a peeling away of the layers of attachments, desires, and limiting beliefs that accumulate over time so that we can ultimately rest in our true essence. Restorative poses teach us not only how to let go but also how to let be.

CONSTRUCTIVE REST POSE

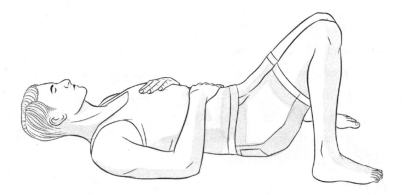

Overview: It might be hard to think of lying on your back as a constructive practice, but studies show that our ability to rest and replenish directly affects our productivity. This pose was given its name by the Alexander Technique and has been adapted by yogis as an integral part of the practice. It is a good place to begin, end, or support your practice from a conscious and intentional space.

How-to: Lie on your back and bend your legs, taking your feet wide and your knees touching. Rest your arms either alongside your body or on your torso, with one hand on your chest and the other hand on your belly. Allow the weight of your body to release down into the support of the floor. Relax your belly, chest, shoulders, and facial muscles. Allow your breath to rise and fall underneath your hands naturally.

Benefits: Physically, this pose aligns the spine, calms the nervous system, and facilities a complete breath. It activates the parasympathetic nervous response, which leads to lower blood pressure, slower brain waves, better digestion, and slower heart rate.

Energetically, this pose is grounding and calming. When we lie on our back, the abdominal muscles can relax, encouraging a deeper breath into the lower belly, which helps to soothe the mind. This is a valuable pose to experience a full, complete breath, balancing the mind and the qualities of *rajas* and *tamas*, bringing us into *satva guna*.

No *bandhas* engaged. Stimulates *prana* and *apana vayu*.

Therapeutic applications: Reduces anxiety, headache, fatigue, lower back pain, and menstrual and menopausal discomfort.

Helpful tip: Place a folded blanket underneath your head if your chin is higher than your forehead.

LEGS UP THE WALL POSE:
VIPARITA KARANI

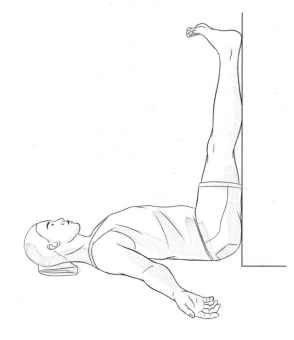

Overview: The literal translation of this pose is the "reversal" (*Viparita*) of "doing" (*Karani*). This profoundly replenishing pose gives us the benefits not only of inverting without putting any pressure on the neck or head but also of being passive. It can be a generous gift we give ourselves at the end of the day or after travel, literally putting our feet up and reversing the flow of gravity.

How-to: Sit on a folded blanket with the right hip flush against the wall and your mat perpendicular to the wall. Have another folded blanket toward the top of the mat for your head to rest on. Slide your left arm and the left side of your torso down the length of the mat and roll onto your back, allowing the right leg, followed by the left leg, to float up against the wall. Adjust your sacrum so that the sit bones rest against the wall and the sacrum evenly releases into the support of the blanket. Slide the folded blanket underneath your head. Float your arms wide, with the elbows bent at a 90-degree angle, palms facing up, and fingertips relaxed. Rest here, allowing the weight of your body to release onto the floor for up to 10 minutes.

Benefits: Physically, Legs Up the Wall pose releases the backs of the legs, the lower back, the chest, the shoulders, and the back of the neck. It brings the deoxygenated blood back to the heart and helps to reduce swelling in the feet.

Energetically, this pose is calming, quieting, and deeply replenishing. It activates the fifth and sixth chakras, facilitating a state of silence, introspection, and inner vision. It also helps us to perceive the world from a new perspective.

Engage *jalandhara bandha.* Stimulates *apana vayu.*

Therapeutic applications: Legs Up the Wall pose alleviates edema, varicose veins, menstrual discomfort, and swollen ankles. Helpful with jet lag and insomnia.

Helpful tips: Wrap a belt or a strap around your thighs to keep your legs together. Place a weighted cushion on your feet to help release the thigh bones into the hip socket. For a hip-opening alternative, bring the soles of your feet together and spread your knees wide apart. If you don't have wall space, practice this pose with a block underneath your sacrum and your legs toward the ceiling.

CORPSE POSE:
SAVASANA

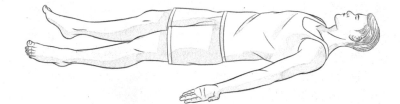

Overview: Corpse pose is one of the most important poses of the Hatha Yoga practice. It is ritualistically practiced at the end of each sequence, representing the final cycle of life, which is destruction. In Corpse pose, we are dismantling our attachment to our body, mind, thoughts, and identity, and learning how to rest in our true essence, which is infinite and unbounded. It transitions us from the act of doing into the art of being.

How-to: Lie on your back with your legs a little wider than hip-distance apart, your feet rolling open, and your arms at a 45-degree angle alongside your body. With your palms facing up, allow your fingertips to curl in toward the palms of your hands naturally. Allow the entire weight of your body to surrender into the support of the floor. Relax each muscle in your body from your toes up to the crown of your head. Rest here for at least 5 minutes in complete stillness.

Benefits: Physically, Corpse pose elicits the parasympathetic nervous response, which, as mentioned earlier, is physiologically healing. It lowers blood pressure, slows down the heart rate, brings blood back to the heart, aids in digestion, and bolsters the immune system.

Energetically, this pose reduces anxiety and facilitates a deep sense of surrender. It activates the seventh chakra, promoting a sense of spiritual awakening and connection to universal intelligence.

No *bandhas* engaged. Stimulates *prana* and *apana vayu*.

Therapeutic applications: This pose is healing for various physical and mental conditions. It aids in blood pressure reduction; alleviates anxiety, lower back pain, fatigue, and chronic pain; and eases overall tension in the body.

Helpful tips: Place a cushion or a rolled-up towel or blanket underneath your knees if you have any lower back pain. If your chin is higher than your forehead, place a folded blanket underneath your head.

AFTERWORD

By *Deepak Chopra*

Where Do You Go from Here?

Royal Yoga has inspired spiritual seekers for many centuries. To help inspire you, we've tried to clear the path of complications and obstacles. I strongly believe that everyday experiences give a glimpse of what it is like to live in the light. I base this belief on one of the most basic principles in Yoga: Consciousness is whole, and we all share in this wholeness. Everyone starts on a level playing field when it comes to awareness. At every moment, you are either aware or not. This is a choice that excludes no one. The light of awareness is universal.

Royal Yoga is more than a set of practices for making you more aware. It offers a vision of the ideal life. This vision also excludes no one because the ideal life is based on consciousness. You can't change what you aren't aware of, and the more aware you are, the greater the changes you can achieve. Humans are the only creatures who can consciously evolve. Yoga is the handbook that shows you how to evolve. The handbook is complete, and whoever you are, its instructions apply to you.

So, if someone asked, "What do I do now?" the one-word answer is

"Evolve." We commonly speak of spiritual seekers, but in reality, there are only spiritual evolvers—or not.

Right now, and in the recent past, I've encountered more people than ever before who have set out on their own spiritual path. They have become inspired by higher consciousness; they've gotten excited about the notion of "Follow your bliss." But a cynic would point out that we have been hearing about the emergence of higher consciousness for at least fifty years, and collective enlightenment still isn't in sight.

Yet there is no reason to be discouraged once you accept a simple but profound truth: Consciousness evolves in a way that fits every individual. Nothing is more individual and fluid. Yet along the path you should be prepared for some highly peculiar, even unique qualities. Here are just a few:

- You can't see the goal in advance.
- You therefore cannot make reliable plans on how to reach the goal.
- Because your inner life is constantly shifting, you never know if your attitude is correct or even if you are equipped for the next phase of the journey.
- Your ego-personality, which supports you in every other activity, is of little use when addressing consciousness. Typically, the ego-personality is an obstacle to, or pulls you away from, any drastic change, particularly if old habits, beliefs, and conditioning are challenged.
- Even though you think and act as an individual, consciousness isn't personal: It's universal, holistic, and, in the end, inconceivable.

All these points have come up in this book, but by gathering them together in one list, I'm giving you the essence of what it feels like to live the vision of Royal Yoga.

Once you recognize that your own evolution must come to terms with everything on this list, the picture changes. The self is transforming the self. You are like a surgeon who wants to perform surgery on himself, which is obviously an impossible task. How can an individual—guided by the ego-personality, which will only sabotage real personal transformation—ever evolve? The answer is not found at the level of the ego or the active mind. Instead, you increasingly let your true unbounded nature come to light; you hold on to the desire to meet your true self, exchanging a series of provisional selves along the way for something everlasting.

These provisional selves, from birth to death and conforming to every situation in between, feel like "I, me, and mine." We own them; we assume we *are* them. But from a Yogic perspective, these selves are just garments to clothe the ego, a superficial covering that masks the true self. Because the true self is the only part of us that knows what is really going on, it invisibly manages our evolution.

Think about an infant facing stages of development that are controlled invisibly from a level of life it has no knowledge of. Ahead lie baby teeth, adult teeth, puberty, the formation of the immune system, the maturation of the brain, and so on. The controller of these processes, we say, is our DNA. But, in fact, the controller is the invisible knowledge encoded in DNA, not the chemical amalgam of a gene, which consists of very ordinary carbon, hydrogen, nitrogen, and oxygen, for the most part.

If there is a similar controller of our conscious evolution, it, too, consists of knowledge. And just as DNA unfolds a child's development on schedule, with a definite time line that puts baby teeth ahead of puberty, the evolution of consciousness unfolds according to a specific time line. But because the whole person is involved, with the inclusion of every personal trait that makes us unique individuals, this silent unfoldment is dynamic, shifting, responsive to life situations, and impossible to predict in advance.

Because the evolution of consciousness is about the entire person at every moment, an inconceivable project is at work, one that is dismantling the setup of separation to arrive at unity consciousness, the true self, Atman, supreme Yoga, or whatever you want to call it. The setup of separation destines you to live in a world of opposites. In the cosmos that we know, and that has shaped every quality of life, evolution is the opposite of entropy. Entropy winds down the universe, like a child's toy whose battery grows weaker until the toy doesn't move anymore. Evolution, like a new battery, reenergizes the universe. Entropy is the force that ensures destruction, and evolution takes the opportunity after each act of destruction to assemble something new from the same ingredients.

Over billions of years, evolution created all living things out of scattered stardust. Yet consider how dust, the simplest ingredient in the universe, led to human DNA, far and away the most complex structure in the universe. On the personal level, evolution proceeds when we dismantle some aspect of the ego-personality so that a more evolved quality can take its place. Destruction is essential, and you must trust that the true self knows better than you do which parts of the darkness must reach the light and when. In Yoga, the all-knowing creative force of Nature is Shakti, the creative intelligence that controls both creation and destruction.

The darkness, being essential, is not to be feared, shunned, or denied. Our strategy as evolving selves is to patiently confront every sign of darkness, accepting that the light will find a way to transform it and reveal the essential truth it hides. There is no need to use the tools of darkness against it, either, since violence, resistance, denial, despair, hatred, and fear are not how the light operates. The light is nothing but awareness revealing something new about itself, enabling the true self, which is universal, to manage everything. A surgeon cannot operate upon himself, but the ego-personality isn't playing the role of a surgeon—the true self plays that role.

Living the vision of Royal Yoga, each of us must remember that the true self is the real self. Only by standing firm in who we really are can the evolution of consciousness take hold every day throughout our lifetime. There's nothing more to know and nothing more to do if you want to live in the light forever.

ACKNOWLEDGMENTS

From Deepak

In recent years, I've developed a passion for Yoga in all its aspects, and I am grateful to my teacher Eddie Stern, whose wisdom and depth of knowledge extend far beyond our daily sessions of practicing Hatha Yoga. No one has ever taught me more about Yoga.

It was inspiring to have Sarah Platt-Finger as my collaborator in this book. She exemplifies all the virtues and benefits of her deep dedication to Yoga.

A writer couldn't be more fortunate than to receive the loyalty, guidance, and personal support of everyone at Harmony Books, beginning with Diana Baroni, whose dedication to publishing is a source of constant admiration. Your insight and decision-making have been crucial in the difficult times we've been passing through—my heartfelt thanks.

I've enjoyed a bond of closeness and shared admiration with my editor, Gary Jansen. You have been wise and tactful beyond anything a writer hopes for. Thanks, too, to the whole Harmony team, including Aaron Wehner, Tammy Blake, Christina Foxley, Marysarah Quinn, Patricia Shaw, Jessie Bright, Andrea Lau, Jessica Heim, Sarah Horgan, and Michele Eniclerico.

My sense of love and caring owes everything to my wife, Rita, and our extended family of children and grandchildren. Thank you for making this journey a shared venture that enriches all of us.

From Sarah Platt-Finger

I would first and foremost like to thank my coauthor, Dr. Deepak Chopra, for the great honor of inviting me to write this book with him. The ecosystem of yoga is vast, with innumerable teachers; it is a great privilege to share my teachings with such a luminary. Thank you for trusting me to be your co-pilot on this project.

To my husband, my spiritual partner, and the person without whom none of the words on my pages would have formed: Yogiraj Alan Finger. Thank you for allowing me to walk alongside you for the past fifteen years, sharing the ISHTA lineage worldwide. Thank you for teaching me everything I know in the process. Your endless support and blessings of this book have meant the world to me.

To Claire Kinsella-Holtje, for reminding me of the power of my own unique voice. I could not have written this book without your mentorship and validation.

To my parents, John and Sheila Platt, who always supported the creative energy within me, even if that meant spending most of my childhood upside down or climbing on the furniture! Thank you for encouraging my words to go on paper from such a young age.

To my sister, Emily, thank you for being my first teacher in life and a role model for life. I am so grateful to you.

Thank you to my editor, Gary Jansen; my publisher, Diana Baroni; and everyone at Penguin Random House, including production editor Patricia Shaw and designer Andrea Lau, for their unwavering support and patience with me. You have made the art of writing a book pure joy and much less daunting than I anticipated! And special thanks to Stephanie Singleton, whose illustrations in this book captivate and celebrate the beauty of the human form through asana.

To my dear friends Alyssa Miller, Mona Anand, Kristin Leal, Loraine Rushton, and Rachel Goldstein. Your sisterhood is my life force energy.

And to my daughter, Satya, for being the light of love and of truth. Because of you, I know I can; and because of you, I always will.

INDEX

ABOUT THE AUTHORS

Deepak Chopra

Deepak Chopra, MD, FACP, founder of the Chopra Foundation (a nonprofit entity for research on well-being and humanitarianism) and Chopra Global (a modern-day health company at the intersection of science and spirituality), is a world-renowned pioneer in integrative medicine and personal transformation. Chopra is a clinical professor of family medicine and public health at the University of California, San Diego, and serves as a senior scientist with Gallup Organization. He is the author of more than ninety books translated into forty-three languages, including numerous *New York Times* bestsellers. *Time* magazine has described Dr. Chopra as "one of the top 100 heroes and icons of the century."

Sarah Platt-Finger

Sarah Platt-Finger is the director of yoga at Chopra Global, and the cofounder of ISHTA Yoga, LLC. Deepak Chopra has called Sarah "an extraordinary teacher of yoga that has called enormously to my well-being." She received her 500-hour certification in the ISHTA lineage in 2004 and was initiated as a yoga master in 2013. Since then, Sarah has made it her life's purpose to share the authentic teachings of yoga worldwide. She believes that the practice of yoga can be used as a microcosm for the reality we create off the mat, and that a deeper awareness of our physical, mental, and emotional patterns can bring us closer to the essence of our being. Sarah teaches an embodied and affirming practice that encourages healing, transformation, and self-empowerment. Always a seeker, she considers motherhood to be her greatest spiritual practice.

Sarah currently lives in Boca Raton, Florida, with her husband, Yogiraj Alan Finger; their daughter, Satya; and their dogs, Malcolm and Thomas. She teaches weekly classes online, pursuing her mission of helping others find a home inside themselves.